"Focus on defusion as a central char important contribution of acceptanc the field of psychotherapy in genera therapist, accustomed to ACT or not, practical advice how to help clients in this direction. Read and learn!"

—**Niklas Törneke, MD**, author of *Learning RFT* and coauthor of *The ABCs of Human Behavior*

"Finally, a book that shows the practitioner how to use defusion in everyday practice. Defusion is perhaps one of the most powerful ingredients in acceptance and commitment therapy (ACT), and one of the most misunderstood. When done well, defusion helps people to overcome unhelpful thinking patterns and direct their energy towards value-consistent living. When done poorly, defusion can be unpleasant and invalidating. *Cognitive Defusion in Practice* shows you how to implement defusion effectively, in a way that helps your clients to feel appreciated and to move through the unhelpful beliefs that seem to interfere with their life. The book includes many clear examples of how to use defusion flexibly, in the full flow of therapy. It is also clearly written and set in the context of evidence and the full ACT model. If you want to learn how to use defusion in a way that helps people to accept themselves and transform their lives, then this book is for you."

—**Joseph Ciarrochi, PhD**, professor at the Institute for Positive Psychology and Education, and coauthor of *The Weight Escape* and *Get Out of Your Mind and Into Your Life for Teens*

Cognitive Defusion

IN PRACTICE

A CLINICIAN'S GUIDE TO
ASSESSING, OBSERVING &
SUPPORTING CHANGE
IN YOUR CLIENT

JOHN T. BLACKLEDGE, PhD

CONTEXT PRESS
An Imprint of New Harbinger Publications, Inc.

Publisher's Note

This publication is designed to provide accurate and authoritative information in regard to the subject matter covered. It is sold with the understanding that the publisher is not engaged in rendering psychological, financial, legal, or other professional services. If expert assistance or counseling is needed, the services of a competent professional should be sought.

Distributed in Canada by Raincoast Books

Copyright © 2015 by John T. Blackledge

        Context Press, An Imprint of New Harbinger Publications, Inc.
        5674 Shattuck Avenue
        Oakland, CA 94609
        www.newharbinger.com

"Carry Your Keys," "Thoughts and Feelings Aren't Causes," and elements of "Slow Speech and Silly Voices" adapted with kind permission from Springer Science+Business Media from *A Practical Guide to Acceptance and Commitment Therapy* by Steven C. Hayes and Kirk D. Strosahl. Copyright © 2004 Steven C. Hayes and Kirk D. Strosahl.

Cover design by Amy Shoup
Acquired by Jess O'Brien
Edited by Ken Knabb

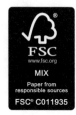 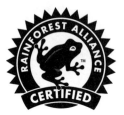

Library of Congress Cataloging-in-Publication Data on file

Printed in the United States of America

17   16   15

10   9   8   7   6   5   4   3   2   1   First printing

For my daughters, Ava and Emma, and my wife, Cyndy.
I love you more than words can express.

Contents

Dear reader,

Welcome to New Harbinger Publications. New Harbinger is dedicated to publishing books based on acceptance and commitment therapy (ACT) and its application to specific areas. New Harbinger has a long-standing reputation as a publisher of quality, well-researched books for general and professional audiences.

As part of New Harbinger's commitment to publishing books based on sound, scientific, clinical research, we oversee all prospective books for the Acceptance and Commitment Therapy Series. Serving as series editors, we comment on proposals and offer guidance as needed, and use a gentle hand in making suggestions regarding the content, depth, and scope of each book.

Books in the Acceptance and Commitment Therapy Series:

- Have an adequate database, appropriate to the strength of the claims being made.

- Are theoretically coherent. They will fit with the ACT model and underlying behavioral principles as they have evolved at the time of writing.

- Orient the reader toward unresolved empirical issues.

- Do not overlap needlessly with existing volumes.

- Avoid jargon and unnecessary entanglement with proprietary methods, leaving ACT work open and available.

- Keep the focus always on what is good for the reader.

- Support the further development of the field.

- Provide information in a way that is of practical use to readers.

These guidelines reflect the values of the broader ACT community. You'll see all of them packed into this book. This series is meant to offer professionals information that can truly be helpful, and to further our ability to alleviate human suffering by inviting creative practitioners into the process of developing, applying, and refining a better approach. This book provides another such invitation.

Sincerely,

Steven C. Hayes, Ph.D., Georg H. Eifert, Ph.D., John Forsyth, Ph.D., and Robyn Walser, Ph.D.

Acknowledgments

First, I would like to thank the members of the ACT community who have come up with so many wonderful defusion techniques over the years. Writing a book such as this is so much simpler when the raw materials have already been assembled and graciously provided. I would especially like to thank Steve Hayes for training and mentoring me over the years, and for encouraging me to target this book at therapists both within and broadly beyond the ACT tradition. Without Steve, I would likely never have found the vitalizing, humanizing, and profound approach to life that is embodied by ACT.

I would also like to thank all the people at New Harbinger for making this book a reality. Acquisitions editor Jess O'Brien and freelance copyeditor Ken Knabb, in particular, provided many excellent editorial suggestions, and did so with great patience. My gratitude also extends to Matt McKay for asking me to write this book in the first place.

Finally, my deepest gratitude goes to my wife, Cyndy, and my daughters, Ava and Emma, for putting up with my anxieties and self-doubts as I attempted to meet deadline after deadline. Their unbounded love, support, and encouragement kept me afloat during this project, as it has throughout the rest of my life. Thank you.

Introduction

This book is intended for psychotherapists interested in learning how to understand and effectively use cognitive defusion in therapy, and perhaps also in their own lives. Defusion, a process by which you learn not to take your thoughts too seriously, plays a central role in acceptance and commitment therapy (ACT; Hayes, Strosahl, & Wilson, 2011). It is most likely that you are reading this book to increase your ability to use defusion in that context. But defusion does not relate only to ACT. The term refers to processes central to any mindfulness-based therapy, and can be used in a wide variety of other treatments. Thus, this book will not just describe how to use defusion in ACT, but how to integrate it into other types of psychotherapy.

For most of us, defusion techniques aren't easy to use at first. One of the core premises of defusion is the assumption that words don't accurately capture reality. This assumption goes against long-held beliefs that there are right and wrong ways to think about things, that words *can* capture absolute truths, and that our problematic thoughts must change for us to become psychologically healthy. Because of these assumptions, it can be difficult to consistently know when or where defusion is appropriate in a therapy session, or in the moment-to-moment flow of our lives. Moreover, many defusion techniques are odd or awkward to use, making it potentially difficult to seamlessly integrate them into a session without creating an exchange that may put off a client. This book will teach you to introduce and use defusion in a variety of ways that make sense to both you and your clients.

The first half of the book (chapters 1–4) describes defusion, discusses its place amongst ACT's other five core processes, provides rationales for using defusion in treatments other than ACT, and discusses several caveats for using defusion effectively and appropriately in any therapeutic context. The second half (chapters 5–10) shows in detail how to use a great variety of different defusion techniques, with comprehensive descriptions of those techniques and sample dialogues that illustrate how to talk about them, even when clients are less than receptive. You will learn several ways to seamlessly introduce defusion to a client for the first time; how to use some helpful defusion metaphors that will give you and your clients accessible ways to understand the concepts that underlie defusion; how to help clients defuse from troublesome thoughts by breaking the rules of language that lead those thoughts to be taken literally; and how to loosen the hold that problematic rules and narratives have on your clients. This book will not only describe how to assess and use defusion in ACT, but also discuss how to integrate it into other types of psychotherapy.

Words are ubiquitous in our lives. They play a critical role in shaping every aspect of what we do, how we view ourselves and our world, and how we feel. Defusion teaches us how to step back from the words—and thus, from the thoughts—that cause us problems; how to take those words and thoughts less seriously. It teaches us how to break free from the verbal corners our thoughts paint us into and how to use our thoughts as tools rather than being used by them, thereby enabling us to live meaningful and vital lives even when our thoughts and our feelings are telling us we can't. It is my most sincere hope that this book will help you do just that, both with yourself and with your clients.

CHAPTER 1

What Is Cognitive Defusion?

Most of us assume that if we have distressing or counterproductive thoughts or feelings, those thoughts and feelings need to change for our lives to get better. We need to "get our thoughts in line," "think more realistically," "get rid of our doubts," or "be level-headed" to act constructively and move ahead. We need to "feel motivated" to get up and move, or to take the edge off our anxiety or sadness if we want to engage the world and live a meaningful life. Assumptions like these are mainstream in most cultures, and even central to psychotherapy's most empirically supported treatments. Most forms of cognitive behavioral therapy make heavy use of cognitive restructuring, a strategy based on the premise that thoughts must change before emotions and overt behavior change. While this assumption is made explicit in cognitive behavioral therapy (CBT), most forms of psychotherapy arguably adopt some version of it as well. How much time do you spend in therapy trying to help your clients think differently about themselves, about their worlds, about their problems? How certain are you that your clients must come to think about things differently for their lives to get better?

No one would argue that it's not nice when our thoughts change for the better, or not easier when our feelings fall in line with what we'd like to be doing. All of us have had experiences where we've been upset about something, only to feel better when we gain a new perspective on it. All of us understand the value of learning to think more logically and rationally about our lives and our world. But you may have noticed that sometimes rational and logical thoughts don't come easy, and that our problematic and distressing thoughts have a way of popping up and sticking around regardless of our efforts to keep them at bay. Cognitive restructuring—or, more generally, learning to think more "accurately" about one's issues—appears to be a viable method of changing human behavior for the better, but it's not the only way. Defusion does not devalue the usefulness of logic and rationality, but it offers additional methods for dealing constructively with problematic thoughts and related emotions.

Cognitive defusion is a relatively new name for a very old process, a process that (as we'll discuss in chapters 2 and 3) is central to acceptance and commitment therapy (ACT; Hayes, Strosahl, & Wilson, 2011) and to a tradition of mindfulness practice that goes back more than two thousand years. The process's original name within ACT—"deliteralization" (Hayes, Strosahl, & Wilson, 1999)—gives a quick sense of what "cognitive defusion" refers to. Normally when we have thoughts, particularly compelling ones, we take them literally. We assume that they capture reality in some fundamental sense, that they perfectly (or perhaps near-perfectly) describe what they purport to describe, and dictate behavior and emotions that are in line with them. We "fuse" with these thoughts, buy into them hook, line, and sinker. We buy into them so thoroughly and so quickly that we likely don't even notice they are thoughts in the first place; we assume that they are simply a reflection of the way things are. To "defuse" from those thoughts means to take them less literally, to "deliteralize" them. (Steven Hayes changed the name from "deliteralization" to "cognitive defusion," because "deliteralization" is pretty hard to say; S. Hayes, personal communication, April 2004.)

This chapter is intended to give you a basic conceptual and experiential understanding of defusion. The "experiential" nature of defusion requires some discussion before we continue. Simply stating that "words don't capture reality" is unlikely to help you defuse from your troublesome thoughts; and, in fact, you might object to the implications of such a simple but far-reaching claim. You need to *experience* how your words (and your thoughts) fail to capture the full breadth and depth of reality; to notice firsthand, moment to moment, the cracks and chinks in the seemingly unassailable wall of words your mind assembles for you. You'll see the experiential, *in vivo* nature of defusion techniques throughout this book, but I'll start in this chapter so that those new to defusion can hopefully get a real sense of what it's like. To facilitate this goal, you are strongly encouraged to take advantage of the online resources mentioned in the "How Does Cognitive Defusion Work?" section, later in this chapter, and to actually do the brief exercises discussed in the following paragraphs as well. First, though, let's talk a little bit more about defusion.

Ultimately, words are nothing more than sounds or scratches on paper. Anyone who has heard a particular foreign language for the first time, or who has seen text written in Sanskrit or Arabic or in Kanji characters (assuming he cannot read such letters and characters) has experienced words in this way. Some words, words that simply describe the physical properties of things, are quite convincing. We can be pretty certain, for example, that when we describe a table as brown and square and wooden that these words correspond pretty well to the reality that is being described. Yet even these kinds of words can fool us into thinking that we fully understand the thing we are describing, that we have captured its essence. It is one thing to know that a table is wooden, and another to actually feel the grain and varying textures of the wood, or see its whorls and luster. It is one thing to hear it is brown, but another to see the exact shade of brown and its variations across the surface.

Words that attempt to evaluate or judge the merit or worth of an object, person, or experience can more deeply fool us into thinking they capture the true essence of what they evaluate. Take a minute or two to recall one of the best moments of your life. Recall that specific experience with as much detail as you can. Remember the sights, the sounds, who was there, what you were doing, what you were feeling. Climb back into that memory and let it play out in front of you. Now imagine the words you would choose to tell someone *exactly* what it was like to experience that moment. Would those words capture the full essence of the experience, or would they fall short? Next, imagine being told by a close friend that someone you just met is a "bad" person. Think how quickly that one word could define the essence of that person, could dramatically alter how you interact with him, could change how you interpret his actions. And yet notice how global the word is, how it pretends to characterize the full range and history of his actions. Notice how it relies on subjective standards that can change from person to person, or even from situation to situation. Notice, in short, how those three little letters create an abstract concept that transforms how you would see and treat that person.

We have come to rely on words so much that we often take them as complete substitutes for the actual experience, person, or thing they refer to. If you watch very young children interacting with a particular object for the first time, for example, you will often see that they pay great attention to its details—what colors it has, what it feels like, what it tastes like, how it responds when it is dropped, and so on. Older children are often simply satisfied to learn the name of a new object, as if knowing the name means they understand exactly what the object is. Recall a conversation with a mental health colleague where she conceptualized a case using a theory you do not subscribe to. She may have given the impression that she was certain that she had articulated the essence of what drove her client's behavior, yet from your point of view it seemed absurd to think that those words could really capture that client's experience. We are most often blinded by our preferred theoretical words when we describe the causes and context of a client's experience. To some extent our words may accurately describe the client's experience, but they may also fall far short of expressing the full breadth and depth of factors that have led that person to think, feel, and act the way he does.

This is not to say that words are not useful. Without words, this book, or any book, would not exist. The vast knowledge of this generation could not be passed on to the next, and indeed this generation would not even have been able to generate that vast knowledge in the first place. Language allows us to create a road map of the world around us, to imagine and create new things, to develop theories of how things work that help us manipulate the world to our advantage. This is the bright side of language, the reason why it has given human beings such a competitive advantage on our planet. Language essentially enables us to categorize, evaluate, and analyze things, to imagine what could and should be, and to take steps to make those coulds and shoulds a reality. Therein lies its usefulness. But there is a dark side to language as well. Once we learn to categorize and evaluate some things, we very quickly try to do the same thing with ourselves and our experiences. My wife and I once did an experiment where we taught children diagnosed with autism how to use the evaluative words "better" and "worse." We started by simply having them apply those words to tangible items like food, drinks, and toys, associating the words with each child's subjective experience of what she preferred and did not prefer. We were very pleased to find, after a few weeks, that many of the children had been spontaneously applying those words to objects not used in the experiment, running around at home and at school saying things like, "This is better than that." But then I wondered how long it would be before they started applying those words to themselves, to others, and to their experiences—"His life is better than mine"; "She's a better person than I am"—with the implication that "I am worse." And, of course, if one is worse than others and has a worse life, that is sufficient cause to feel emotions like embarrassment, shame, sadness, anxiety, or jealousy, with all the particular problems those emotions can evoke.

All of us do that with words. In particular, we appear to have a tremendous ability to evaluate things in a negative way. Take a minute to look around the room and see if you can find anything (or anyone) that you cannot evaluate negatively in some way. Recall how often you have had critical thoughts about others, or yourself, or your job, or your life. Think of the times your clients have looked at themselves and their lives and evaluated them as "lacking," as "flawed," as different from what they "should" be. Think of the times when you have done this with your own life. Language has turned us into evaluative and categorical machines with no "off-switch" and no target off-limits. Sometimes this works well enough for us, but at other times believing that such words capture the essence of reality can cause great pain and great dysfunction.

From a therapeutic perspective, there are different ways to try to address the damage caused by words. A common way, exemplified both in everyday culture and more systematically and comprehensively in conventional cognitive behavior therapy, is to try to change the words that are causing problems into more logical and factually accurate ones. Another way is to learn to take words, or thoughts, less seriously, to realize experientially that words (particularly the evaluative and prescriptive ones) cannot capture the truth, and thus do not need to be changed or heeded. This latter method, first referred to as "cognitive defusion" in print by Hayes and Strosahl (2004), is the topic of this book. As it turns out, however, the process referred to by that phrase has been around for a lot longer than a decade.

A Brief History of Cognitive Defusion

"In the sky there is no distinction of east and west; people create distinctions out of their own minds and then believe them to be true."

—Siddhartha Gautama (Buddha)

Anyone who has cultivated a meditation practice likely knows the experience of noticing a thought simply as a thought, rather than as a binding reality. While the term "cognitive defusion" is new and includes some refinements and expansions, the process it generally refers to has been recognized for millennia. Fletcher and Hayes (2005) analyzed the notion of mindfulness, central both to Buddhism and to a new wave of empirically supported mindfulness-based cognitive behavioral therapies such as acceptance and commitment therapy (ACT; Hayes, Strosahl, & Wilson, 2011), mindfulness-based cognitive therapy (Segal, Williams, & Teasdale, 2002), and dialectical behavior therapy (Linehan, 1993). They concluded that mindfulness represents the confluence of four interrelated psychological processes: acceptance of one's experience as it is, increased contact with the present moment, a sense of self-as-context or "transcendent sense of self" (Fletcher & Hayes, p. 321), and cognitive defusion. Aspects of the notion of defusion have even shown up in other areas of empirical psychology. Jakobovits and Lambert (1961), for example, coined the phrase "semantic satiation" to refer to a word's subjective loss of meaning after the word has been repeated over and over, a phenomenon first researched by Severance and Washburn (1907).

But while the term "semantic satiation" refers to a single technique that leads to deliteralization, and mindfulness evokes a relatively limited set of techniques (meditation, mindfulness, and perhaps the use of koans), cognitive defusion refers to any technique or practice that results in a temporary loss or weakening of word meaning, or at least to a weakening of the power words hold over subsequent behavior. Why is this distinction important for a psychotherapist? Because it means that a whole host of different techniques can be used to promote defusion from problematic thoughts in therapy. If one technique does not work with a particular client, or the client refuses to use it, then other techniques can be brought to bear. A good number of ACT therapists, and sometimes their clients, have even invented new defusion techniques, allowing therapists to use defusion techniques that fit their personal styles.

How Does Cognitive Defusion Work?

For words to carry meaning, they must be experienced in a particular context. As an example, say the word "milk" aloud once, and notice what comes to mind when you focus on the word. Can you see a glass of milk? Can you feel the coldness of the glass in your hand, or imagine how the milk tastes? Did you think of a cow or a milk carton, or (if you dislike milk or are allergic to it) experience a sense of disgust? When experienced under normal conditions, words have the power to evoke such sensations, images, and emotions.

Now, before reading the next paragraph, say the word "milk" out loud quickly for at least thirty seconds.

Toward the end of that thirty seconds, it is unlikely that you were experiencing any of the sensations or images that showed up when you said the word just once. Instead, you were probably focused on the oddness of the sound coming out of your mouth, or even the physical sensations of producing that sound in your throat and your mouth. By changing the context in which you experienced the word (in this case, repeating it over and over), the meaning of the word was temporarily lost. And even though the loss of meaning was temporary (you can now likely say the word "milk" once and experience all the familiar sensations and images associated with it), an important lesson can be learned from the exercise. Spoken words are simply sounds and the physical sensations involved with producing those sounds. When you speak or hear a word under normal conditions, the word has the power to bring sensations and images of things into the room that actually are not even there, to induce emotions that otherwise would not arise. But when you experience words under abnormal conditions, you start to realize how "fishy" they are, how they have the illusory power to create experiences out of thin air.

To bring this experience even closer to home, think of an issue you have been struggling with, and distill it down to one word that captures much of its potency. Say that word out loud once and notice the sensations, images, emotions, and thoughts that come up. Now, say the word over and over quickly for thirty seconds, and notice if your experience changes. As you will see in chapter 10, repeated experiments using this simple technique have suggested that it can have potent effects in changing how words function, and perhaps even a lasting effect on how we perceive our troublesome thoughts in general. Fortunately, there are also many other parameters of language use that can be violated (in other words, many different contextual features that can be changed) to help us experience language in a defused manner.

Grammatical Conventions

As you have probably noticed from modern-day texting, grammar and spelling do not have to be perfect in order for a sentence to convey the indicated meaning. But there are limits. The "milk" exercise demonstrates one limit. A word is normally only said once, not multiple times in a row. Violation of this language convention causes the word to function in a different manner. Additionally, words must be ordered in a particular fashion for a sentence to convey meaning. For example, the veracity of a troublesome thought like "No matter what I do in life, I fail" could be experienced a bit more tentatively if reordered as "life, fail No I in I matter what do." (An automatic sentence scrambler can be found online using the search term "sentence scramble generator.") Written words must also be spelled reasonably correctly to convey the proper meaning. To experience the effects of violating this convention firsthand, do an online search for "text mechanic," select the appropriate link, and then click on the "Word Scrambler/Descrambler" button. Type in a thought about your life, preferably one that elicits relatively strong affect. Before and after "scrambling" all the words in the sentence, read it carefully and notice your experience.

The rate of speech must also be relatively moderate for words to convey meaning. Imagine, for example, listening to an auctioneer and trying to decipher what is being said. A similar effect occurs when speaking at a very slow rate, especially when each syllable is elongated. And it goes without saying that one must understand the meaning of a word for the word to carry meaning. One way to violate this language convention is to translate one or more key words in a troublesome thought to a foreign language that one does not speak. For example, using an online tool like Google Translate to get a partial Czech-language translation of "I am a bad person" yields "I am a spatny person," a sentence that can help highlight the arbitrary nature of words.

Style of Speech

When thoughts are spoken, the manner in which they are spoken typically matches the gravity or lightness of the thought's content. Serious thoughts about one's sadness, for example, are typically spoken in a relatively (but not overly) slow, grave manner. Thoughts conveying anger are typically spoken in a loud, emphatic, relatively rapid style. Speaking a thought in a manner highly incongruent with its content violates this convention. In ACT, a variety of different ways of accomplishing this effect have been used. A client might be asked to sing a troubling thought in an operatic voice, or to sing the words to a melody of an upbeat song. Or one could speak the thought while imitating a character such as Donald Duck, or Mickey Mouse, or any character with a very unusual voice. The wedding scene from the movie *The Princess Bride* (viewable on YouTube with the search terms "princess bride marriage") illustrates this well. In the video clip, a priest is delivering a wedding speech in a comedic tone of voice, undercutting the seriousness with which such speeches are typically made. While the tone does not make the words lose meaning, it does make the listeners respond quite differently than they would if the words had been spoken in the conventional manner.

Focus on the Content of Language

When we speak with meaning or listen with understanding, our attention is focused on the content of what is being said or thought. Once we begin to focus on the process of producing or hearing the words, or begin to notice thoughts as thoughts, words start to lose meaning. During many types of formal sitting meditation, the meditator is instructed to focus on the breath and to notice (and perhaps label as "thinking") any thoughts that arise, without attempting to change or control them. Over time, this leads the meditator to notice the illusory quality of thoughts and become less bound by their meanings. Noticing the process of thoughts arising rather than fixating on their content helps achieve this result. Alternately, you may have had the experience of stumbling over the pronunciation of a word or even failing to recognize a very familiar word, and have noticed that the word's meaning temporarily disappears. A rather irreverent example of this version of focusing on process versus content occurs in a road scene clip from the movie *Black Sheep*, where both characters (under the influence of marijuana) perseverate over the pronunciation of the word "road."

A More Technical Account of Cognitive Defusion

Many definitions for defusion (deliteralization), of varying degrees of specificity, have been proposed in the past twenty years. Most recently, Hayes and colleagues (2011) stated that fusion (the opposite of defusion) involves "the pouring together of verbal/cognitive processes and direct experience such that the individual cannot discriminate between the two" (p. 244). This often results in a "verbal dominance in behavioral regulation" (p. 69) that establishes thoughts as a substitute for direct experience, and can lead us to believe problematic or inaccurate thoughts without even referencing or monitoring the experiences they claim to capture. Hayes and colleagues (2012) note that this can often lead to an overadherence to verbal rules that describe how we should and should not behave, resulting in the repetition of such rule-governed behaviors even when the indicated behaviors are ineffective or lead to undesirable consequences. A similar result occurs with respect to language that evaluates (often negatively) ourselves, the world, and the people around us. Once we believe such evaluations, we act in ways that are consistent with them. If we conflate those evaluations with actual direct experience, we may cease to consistently check in with our direct experiences to see how concordant those evaluations and experiences are.

But why do thoughts come to achieve such dominant importance in the first place? Hayes and colleagues (2012) believe it comes down to context.

Language is an extremely useful tool. The verbal rules that we generate, or that are handed down to us from textbooks, parents, or teachers, are often very useful. We are consistently expected to have good verbal reasons for why we behave the way we do, even if those verbal reasons are not "true." (For example, if you state that you cannot come to work because you are sick, your employer may excuse you even if you are not really sick.) These nearly omnipresent contextual factors—usefulness and a demand for verbal reason-giving and verbal coherence—encourage an overreliance on language. The more detailed contextual aspects of language use discussed earlier in this chapter (involving, for example, grammatical conventions and style of speech; see Blackledge, 2007, for a more technical account) combine with these factors to produce literal belief in our thoughts.

Defusion, then, involves a variety of interventions that counter this overreliance on language and the damage it can cause. Refining the largely experiential and hopefully accessible treatment of defusion presented earlier in this chapter, Hayes and colleagues (2012) state that "defusion does not eliminate verbal meaning—it just reduces its automatic effect on behavior such that other sources of behavioral regulation can better participate in the moment" (p. 245). These alternative sources of behavioral regulation involve an increased awareness of directly experienced, moment-to-moment cues and consequences providing essential data regarding the effectiveness of our actions that can then be used to redirect our efforts. Another source of pertinent behavioral regulation is the realization that, since thoughts are not binding, one can choose which thoughts are helpful and which are not, and act accordingly. Thus, pragmatism plays an important role in helping us decide when to believe or not believe our thoughts. If you find it troubling that the veracity of a thought could essentially come down to personal preference or simple workability, you are not alone. The very important issue of finding meaning and ethical, prosocial behavior amidst defusion will be discussed in detail in chapter 4.

Conclusion

Defusion stands as an alternative to cognitive restructuring or to the more general notion of "having to think accurately about things." It's an alternative that allows problematic or distressing thoughts to arise without functioning in problematic ways. Defusion does this experientially, by breaking the rules of language use in ways that expose language's inability to capture the full depth of our experiences, to describe our lives and our world with perfect accuracy. While it is a central component in ACT, it has long been part of the mindfulness tradition, and can be used in a wide variety of psychotherapeutic treatments. These latter issues will be discussed in detail in chapters 3 and 4. Chapter 10 will review empirical evidence for defusion's effects.

CHAPTER 2

The Role of Cognitive Defusion in Acceptance and Commitment Therapy

While the process appears to be transferable to other forms of psychotherapy, cognitive defusion plays an integral role in acceptance and commitment therapy (ACT; see, for example, Hayes, Strosahl, & Wilson, 2011). Whether you are using defusion from an ACT perspective or not, understanding how it interacts with other therapeutic processes can facilitate a more strategic, focused use.

The Components of Psychological Flexibility

The overarching goal of ACT is increased psychological flexibility, which is defined as "contacting the present moment as a conscious human being, fully and without defense, as it is and not as what it says it is, and persisting or changing in behavior in the service of chosen values" (Hayes, Pistorello, & Levin, 2012, p. 985). In this section I will examine the nature of the subprocesses of psychological flexibility, and then discuss how defusion plays a critical role in facilitating each of them.

Values

The primary aim of ACT is to increase a person's ability to act consistently with her chosen values. The term "values," however, has a markedly different connotation than it typically carries. In ACT, values are ways of behaving that bring increased meaning, purpose, and vitality to an individual. More technically, they are "freely chosen, verbally constructed consequences of ongoing, dynamic, evolving patterns of activity, which establish predominant reinforcers for that activity that are intrinsic in engagement in the valued behavioral pattern itself" (Wilson & DuFrene, 2009, p. 66). The "freely chosen" aspect of values in ACT highlights a primary way in which the ACT meaning differs from the more common understanding of the term, as clients are guided to choose values that they truly hold, independent of what they "should" value or what others value. Values are "verbally constructed consequences" in that the client verbally clarifies, in various domains of functioning, both how she would like her life to look and individual behaviors and qualities of action that are consistent with or likely to lead to such outcomes. For example, in the domain of parenting, you might value striving for a trusting, supportive, loving, and caring relationship, and clarify a number of specific behaviors you could engage in that convey those qualities and are likely, over the long term, to produce such a relationship. Other typical ACT values domains include intimate relationships, spirituality, education or career, and friendships.

Values consist of "ongoing, dynamic, evolving patterns of activity," in that they reflect a potentially large number of specific behaviors or activities that are thematically related, that reflect the essence of their stated parameters, and that might change over time. For example, a person with a spiritual value of being actively engaged with the world, other people, and nature could act out this value in a variety of ways. He could prompt himself to be fully present when going about daily activities, take time to walk in the woods regularly, try to show up with a sense of connection when talking with others, make efforts to genuinely empathize with those who are suffering, help his neighbors, and so on. Over time, he might find additional ways of expressing this value.

The designated "outcome" of a value, such as being a loving, supportive, and caring parent, is never ultimately and permanently achieved. In fact, the desired consequences of behavior consistent with a value may sometimes seem rather distant. Building a loving, supportive, and caring relationship takes a lot of time, effort, and consistency, and the benefits of building one might seem far in the future. But the sense of supportiveness, lovingness, and caring may also arise immediately while you engage in moment-to-moment behaviors consistent with this value, especially when you are aware of the connection between the value and the behaviors that demonstrate it. In other words, values "establish predominant reinforcers…that are intrinsic in engagement in the valued behavioral pattern itself." Values are lived out in individual moments, and the benefits of acting consistently with them can, at least at times, be immediately realized.

Commitment

Commitment, or committed action, "is a values-based action that occurs at a particular moment in time and that is deliberately linked to creating a pattern of action that serves the value" (Hayes et al., 2011, p. 328). The term "commitment" most obviously refers to a verbal vow to engage is some behavior or set of behaviors at a future time. Although this orientation toward the future can be a component of a commitment in ACT, such commitment also involves the actual act of engaging in behaviors consistent with a chosen value. This way of looking at commitment highlights the moment-to-moment nature of valued living in ACT, and also implies that in each new moment you can make the choice to act consistently with a given value or not, regardless of how you behaved the moment before.

Acceptance

Acting consistently with values is hard. Being a patient, loving, supportive, and caring parent, for example, is all well and good. But behaving consistently with such a value in the middle of a long, stressful work week when time is short and your children are misbehaving can be very challenging. Anxiety, frustration, anger, fatigue, and a whole host of unpleasant emotions may arise. To engage in valued living and reap the rewards, you must persist in the face of such distress. Unfortunately, this is much easier said than done. Understandably, most forms of psychotherapy attempt to reduce or eliminate this distress, and perhaps most psychotherapeutic theories assume that distress must be reduced or eliminated in order for a vital and meaningful life to be lived.

At the core of ACT, however, is the assumption that attempts to eliminate psychological distress will ultimately be ineffective, and even, at times, counterproductive. From this perspective, it is the nature of life to cause distress even under normal circumstances, and avoiding sizeable degrees of distress (from losses of loved ones, illness, thwarted plans and desires, day-to-day stress, and so on) becomes untenable. Thus, the ACT therapist attempts to help the client accept unpleasant feelings, thoughts, and other experiences that arise when problems in valued living present themselves. As with values, the term "acceptance" carries some misleading connotations that, in this case, might lead you to think the client should "just get over it," "toughen up," "grin and bear it," and so on. But Hayes and colleagues (2011) offer formal definitions of both acceptance and willingness that differ markedly from these connotations. From their perspective, acceptance "is the adoption of an intentionally open, receptive, flexible, and nonjudgmental posture with respect to moment-to-moment experience" (p. 77). Thus, to accept distress, you allow it to arise when it arises, experience what is there to be experienced, and do not buy into the host of negative evaluations that typically accompany unpleasant emotions and experiences.

Willingness, often used as a synonym for acceptance in ACT, highlights the connection between acceptance and commitment to values-based action. Willingness is defined as "the voluntary and values-based choice to enable or sustain contact with private experiences or the events that will likely occasion them" (Hayes et al., 2011, p. 77). This definition highlights the fact that acceptance is used strategically in ACT. Many have noticed similarities between ACT and Buddhism, from which ACT has borrowed premises, perspectives, and meditative techniques. (For a discussion of the similarities and differences between ACT and Buddhism, see Hayes, 2002.) In Buddhism, full and ongoing acceptance of one's experience is an explicit, albeit intermediate, goal on the path to enlightenment. In ACT, acceptance is used to facilitate valued living when distress arises.

Present-Moment Awareness

An increased awareness of the present moment is fostered in ACT for several different reasons. First, an acceptance of your experience directly implies an acceptance of what is being experienced *here and now*. Worrisome thoughts about the future, feelings of guilt about past actions, or imminent anxiety or sadness are all experienced now, and counterproductive attempts to avoid them also occur now. It follows that attempts to enact new ways of responding to these thoughts and other experiences (involving, for example, ACT-based acceptance and defusion strategies) must also occur in the here and now.

Second, real-world contingencies for behavior also occur in the here and now. If we wish to respond with maximal effectiveness to what is happening around us, we need to be aware of these contingencies. There is, of course, a place for planning and strategizing; but no plan will work if it does not address the current realities of the time and place it is applied to. Awareness of present-moment contingencies facilitates both problem solving and values-driven action (though the two are often one and the same). Given the vast range of values-consistent behaviors that can emerge, opportunities to engage in them can easily be overlooked if we remain "stuck in our heads" and unaware of what is happening before us.

Present-moment awareness intersects with values in another way. A frequent aspect of values-consistent behavior appears to be vitality—an experience of being fully in the moment and feeling fully alive. This certainly does not always happen when engaging in valued living, but detailed reflection on some of the best moments of our lives (moments when we were doing things that really mattered to us) typically reveals a marked in-the-moment quality.

Self-as-Context

Normally we do not recognize our thoughts as thoughts. Instead, we tend to see them as 100% factual reflections of reality. When self-referential thoughts are viewed from this perspective, the content of the thoughts appears to define who we are as people. When viewed from a similar perspective, emotions can appear self-definitional as well. A person who frequently experiences anxiety might describe himself as an "anxious person," as if "anxious" fully and completely defines him. A person experiencing a deep sadness at the loss of a loved one might not only think of herself as a "sad person," but she might feel like the sadness will always remain, as if she were viewing the world through a pair of gray-colored glasses that seem destined to permanently color her experiences. When thoughts and emotions appear to define who we are as people, or when we are so caught up with thoughts and emotions that we can see little else in our experience, we are said to be experiencing a sense of *self-as-content* (see, for example, Hayes et al., 2011, pp. 81–84). When the content that is being experienced is negative, such a sense of self can be especially debilitating. In such cases, avoidance of your experience, and thus a relative lack of values-driven behavior, can become increasingly likely.

An antidote for a dysfunctional sense of self-as-content involves developing a sense of *self-as-context*. Hayes and colleagues (2011) noted that "the psychological literature contains numerous terms and concepts that allude to this aspect of self: a transcendent sense of self, the observing self, noticing self, continuity of consciousness, pure consciousness, pure awareness, and others" (p. 85). Essentially, adopting a sense of self-as-context involves noticing your thoughts and feelings as changing experiences that you have, rather than self-definitional things that can threaten your integrity and existence; in other words, noticing the "part of you" that notices your thoughts and feelings, and noticing that that part of you remains a constant that is always available to observe your changing thoughts and feelings and their waxing and waning intensities.

The experience described here may appear overly philosophical, but the genesis of such a sense of self can, and has been, described in psychological terms (see, for example, Kohlenberg & Tsai, 1991, pp. 128–139; see also Hayes et al., 2011, pp. 85–86). To shift to first person for a moment: Since the time I began learning language, I have been bombarded with questions about what *I* want, what *I* am thinking or feeling, where *I* was at some point in the past or will be in the future, what *I* see or hear, and so on. I, like you, have probably heard tens of thousands of such questions over my middle-aged lifetime, most of which have had widely varying answers. The one constant in these questions and answers has been the perspective from which *I* have wanted, thought, felt, been, seen, and heard everything *I* have experienced. Everything I have experienced, I have experienced from that same place, that same locus of perspective. Though the content of my experiences can change vastly from moment to moment, I always experience it from right here, right now. This ubiquitous "I" is thus an essential part of the context in which everything is experienced—it defines who I unvaryingly am as a person. "I" am the context in which my thoughts, feelings, and sensations are experienced. The experiencing of a sense of self-as-context, then, involves discerning the stable and enduring "I" that observes the transient ebb and flow of my thoughts, emotions, sensations, and memories—and noticing those experiences, moment to moment, from that unchanging "observer perspective" (Hayes et al., 2011, p. 66).

The ability to slide into such a sense of self-as-context can have significant benefits. Aside from being closely related to the ability to understand others' perspectives and to develop empathy (see, for example, McHugh & Stewart, 2012), adopting a sense of self-as-context appears to facilitate acceptance of, and a more productive response to, difficult thoughts, memories, emotions, and other experiences. If a distressing thought or emotion is not viewed as self-defining (and thus potentially self-destroying or self-damaging), it can become less threatening and thus more readily accepted. If the ebb and flow of thoughts and feelings can be seen at least periodically from an observer perspective, then it comes to be understood that perhaps thoughts and feelings are not as permanent and not as threatening as they once appeared to be. And if a distressing thought can be viewed from a distance rather than held tightly and believed unquestioningly, that thought may begin to lose some of its power.

Those exposed to ACT can often have a difficult time understanding the conceptual differences between defusion and self-as-context and determining which techniques are intended to facilitate defusion and which are intended to instill a sense of self-as-context. Part of the difficulty arises because use of either set of techniques inevitably leads to *both* defusion and a sense of self-as-context. The classic "Milk" defusion exercise you were asked to conduct in chapter 1, for example, very readily breaks up the literal meaning of the word and embodies what defusion can be. But the exercise also shapes a distinction between the sounds and physical sensations associated with the word "milk" and the "you" who is noticing those sounds and sensations. ACT's classic "Observer" exercise (where clients are asked to repeatedly notice the distinction between their thoughts, feelings, and physical sensations and the "observer you" who is noticing them) instills a sense of self-as-context. But the distance gained from thoughts in that exercise also works to erode their pervasive, self-defining literality. In other words, when you experience a sense of self-as-*content*, you are relatively fused with the thoughts you are having. You both take them literally and do not notice the distinction between those thoughts and the "you" that is noticing them. When you experience a sense of self-as-*context*, you gain a psychological distance from your thoughts that helps you take them less literally. Because both processes refer directly to changing the relationship you have to your thoughts in similar ways, both produce similar outcomes.

From an ontological standpoint, the conceptual overlap between defusion and self-as-context could perhaps be considered problematic, but not if (in the spirit of defusion) the constructs are not viewed as absolute, discrete truths. We have a multifaceted relationship with our thoughts and feelings. From an applied psychology perspective in particular, it makes sense to have terms that highlight those different facets and explicitly remind therapists what specific kinds of changes we are trying to produce in our clients and the kinds of techniques deemed most likely to produce them. Self-as-context interventions are primarily intended to showcase the ever-changing nature and intensity of your thoughts, feelings, and sensations; to demonstrate that they do not define you as a human being; and to highlight the distinction between you as an observer and the psychological content you observe. Defusion interventions are primarily intended to undermine the literal meanings and functions of problematic thoughts. In the end, both help you get more distance from those problematic thoughts and narratives and take them less seriously. In practice, it's not important for an ACT therapist to know precisely where one process "ends" and the other "begins," as if they were real things with distinct boundaries. Rather, it is important simply to know how to use self-as-context techniques and exercises to help clients step into that observer perspective when they are struggling, and how to use defusion techniques to help them take problematic thoughts less seriously.

Cognitive Defusion in Action: Defusion and Core ACT Processes

Defusion interacts in multiple, critical ways with the five psychological processes discussed above. Considering that most (if not all) of these processes are not unique to ACT, awareness of these interactions can be helpful whether you are using defusion strategies in a pure ACT context or not.

Acceptance and Defusion

From an ACT perspective, language can dramatically alter how we perceive and react to emotions and other experiences. Imagine, for example, how a cat might respond to being "ambushed" by another cat it shares a home with. It would likely experience something similar to anxiety or fear, and respond overtly by running or fighting back. It would also likely be agitated for a few minutes following disengagement of the attack, but then return to its usual routine of calmly preening and sleeping. In contrast, imagine a fully verbal human returning home and being ambushed by a housemate. She would no doubt experience the same fear and fight-or-flight reactions the cat exhibited, but much more would likely be added. She might have lingering anxiety and discomfort, based in part on thoughts like "Home is no longer safe," or "What did I do to deserve this?" This could lead to an increased avoidance of home. Based on what we know about trauma, the anxiety and avoidance could become generalized, accompanied by thoughts such as "The world is no longer safe," "I have to be vigilant at all times to prevent this from happening again," and so on. Additional evaluative thoughts might follow and add to the distress: "Something's very wrong with me." "This stress is unbearable." "I can't trust anyone." "My life is a complete mess." The cat would be unburdened by thoughts like this. The person might be virtually disabled.

Asking any human being to accept his experiences as defined literally by the content of thoughts such as these would be cruel, as well as unrealistic. Either the thoughts must change, or the person's faith in the sanctity of thoughts must be shaken. Defusion plays a profound role in facilitating acceptance of distressing experiences because it works to deliteralize language, to help us see thoughts as thoughts rather than as definitive commentaries on our experiences. The scenario described above involves not just the distressing experiences of anxiety, fight or flight, and situational alertness that would be prompted by the presence of an assaultive housemate. It also involves layers of verbalizations that broaden and intensify the scope of the threat; that cause us to negatively evaluate ourselves, others, and the world; that place perceived limits on what can be tolerated and the behaviors that we "must" or "cannot" now engage in. If these layers can be exposed for what they are, using techniques similar to those in chapter 1 and most of the rest of this book, the core experience and the many, many words that accompany it can be more humanely accepted. Not easily accepted by any means, though even that sometimes happens (as indicated by the results of many of the defusion studies summarized in chapter 10). But the thicket you are standing in can be at least temporarily dethorned, perhaps long enough to allow you to turn some attention toward the horizon and to take steps through the branches and boughs toward it.

As suggested above, defusion is at times brought to bear on general thoughts about the toxicity or bearableness of unpleasant emotions, about what their presence says about us as people or about life in general, and about what is and is not possible when they are present. Many of us, even as psychotherapists, may hold the implicit or explicit assumption that the willing experience of too much "negative" emotion is dangerous or beyond bearing. Certainly, things like experiencing repeated panic attacks when you have a heart condition are a source for concern. But does the intermittent full experiencing of strong emotions that are largely there already (and that often accompany a variety of dysfunctional or counterproductive responses to them) damage us irreparably or become *literally* unbearable? And does this full experiencing of such emotions really harm us when we do it willingly in order to engage something that matters deeply to us? Verbal cases for and against the possibility could be made, but the point is that successfully used defusion strategies can soften your belief in the feared possibility enough to try and see what actually happens.

A similar possibility exists with negative evaluations about ourselves and others, and how the "realities" pointed to by those thoughts limit our behavior and our possibilities. An unpleasant emotion may seem unacceptable, in part, because our minds convince us that the presence of that emotion precludes certain actions and forces others. High anxiety in a person who values social contact, for example, may come with thoughts that state that social interaction is too dangerous and avoidance is the only option. Such emotions become more acceptable when you can defuse from such prescriptive and proscriptive thoughts, experiencing what is there to be experienced and engaging in what matters.

Verbal evaluations play another important role relevant to acceptance that defusion can address. Acceptance can easily come to be viewed as the "right" thing to do and avoidance the "wrong" thing to do. This may cause us to verbally evaluate ourselves as "weak," "lazy," "hopeless," and so on at times when we avoid rather than accept our difficult experiences. In other words, we may believe that we "have to" accept unpleasant experiences, and that there is "something wrong" with us when we do not. Believing such thoughts contributes to a cycle of debilitating negative self-evaluation that may already be fueling problematic avoidance and a lack of values-driven action. Acceptance is a choice that can be made or not made at any given moment. Thoughts that pretend to evaluate that choice from some supposedly objective and binding perspective are simply thoughts.

Values and Defusion

Defusion can assist with a similar set of evaluative thoughts that arises when your values have been clarified. It is especially easy to verbally frame values-consistent behavior as "good" and inconsistent behavior as "bad," in part because living with increased meaning, purpose, and vitality is quite desirable. Given this propensity, chastising yourself for not making values-driven choices becomes a very tangible risk. Doing so can certainly serve as an effective motivation to make more values-driven choices. However, as Wilson and Murrell (2004) have noted, "aversive stimuli…generate a sharp narrowing of behavioral response patterns" (p. 128), meaning that behavior driven primarily by the avoidance of aversive stimuli (such as negative self-evaluations and the emotions they engender) can all too often lead to inflexible and potentially problematic behavior. For this reason, defusion may be used to cut through "good" and "bad" evaluations of values-driven behavior and help the client to view valued living as simply a moment-to-moment choice. Workability becomes the ultimate criterion. Simply put, does your life work better when you act consistently with values? If so, then you can choose to act consistently with a value in the next moment. Defusion can then be brought to bear on thoughts that critique the "idiocy" of acting inconsistently with values and that lead to counterproductive behavior.

Verbal rules about how you "must" or "must not" pursue given values can cause difficulty as well. As an example, when I was an adolescent, I had a rather rigid set of rules regarding how to pursue a romantic relationship. I would keep a respectful distance (with an emphasis on "distance" and a definition of "respect" that functionally gave no hint that I was romantically interested), and then give the young woman a letter detailing how I thought and felt about her. These efforts were ineffective and, quite frankly, odd, yet I repeated them because that was the way I thought I was supposed to do it. But successful pursuit of a romantic relationship requires flexible behavior— attention to moment-to-moment verbal and nonverbal cues, timely provision of cues that reflect your intentions, reciprocation, and typically a graded expression of interest. Rigid adherence to thoughts about how I was "supposed to" behave to further a value blinded me to direct feedback about what was and was not working for others. This same rigid rule governance occurs in many areas of our lives. Perhaps most often, we simply continue to do things in a certain way because that is the way we have always done them, or that is the way we are "supposed to" do them, or simply because we have not considered alternatives. Defusion can be used to help highlight and unhook from potentially ineffective rules. It can even be used to help sift through the consequences of doing something different or unconventional (for example, thoughts about the "danger" of doing something that might lead to embarrassment or disapproval).

At times, particularly philosophical clients who have learned defusion's take-home message may start to question the veracity of their own values. If words have "no meaning," or at least cannot fully capture direct experience, then doesn't that mean your values have no meaning? A focus on workability and direct experience is useful here. What is your direct experience of what your life is like when you live consistently with your values? Do you feel more alive? Does your life feel more meaningful, more purposeful? What if those direct experiences are the measure of what matters to you, rather than a purely verbal evaluation? At times like this, it is important to remember that part of the lesson of defusion is not that there is no meaning in life, but simply that what is most meaningful often cannot be fully described in words. Thus, the thought "Life has no meaning" is simply another set of problematic words to unhook from.

At times, the specific actions you associate with values can take on an illusory all-or-nothing quality. A colleague once reported that, in the months leading up to his father's death, he made meaningful and effective efforts to reconcile with and grow closer to him. His father was a Vietnam war veteran and had suffered greatly from the experience, which contributed toward a contentious relationship between him and his children. My colleague was clear about wanting to be closer with his father and about honoring what his father had been through and what he found to be important, but his father's death appeared to cut those plans short. Nevertheless, he managed to find an interesting and creative way to continue his effort to honor his father. His father's truck, painted orange with a black "agent orange" insignia and a black-and-white POW/MIA banner, had always been a symbol of the distance between him and his father. Now, he drove his father's truck regularly to work at a psychological treatment center, explaining to clients who wondered why their therapist drove such a truck that it made him feel closer to his father and more accepting and honoring of him.

You could imagine a similar scenario playing out with an avid hiker and climber who lost the use of his legs. It would be all too easy for such a person to assume that his recreational values—being outdoors, connecting with nature, challenging himself physically and mentally, throwing himself into the moment—could no longer be lived. But to put it more bluntly than you would prudently say it to a person in this position, challenge, connection to nature, and being in the moment can still be experienced in a wheelchair. In both the case of the man who lost his father and the man who lost the use of his legs, there would be a great degree of sadness and loss that would need to be acknowledged and some very difficult thoughts about unfairness, hopelessness, and so on to unhook from in order to embrace what could still be done. But defusion can help us find the humanity, vitality, meaning, and opportunities to act that exist between the cracks of extremely difficult situations and the narratives our minds weave about them.

Commitment and Defusion

Commitment can also easily take on an "all or nothing" quality, especially when you have behaved in a manner that is clearly inconsistent with your values. At such moments it can be easy to fuse with thoughts that you have "blown it" and can no longer engage in any relevant values-driven actions. As an example, a colleague had "burned his bridges" with his adult daughter as a result of a series of deeply regretted life choices. After reorienting himself, he realized that he very much valued a closer relationship with her, but few (if any) options seemed open. He chose to contact his daughter a couple of times a year and tell her that he would love to see her again, and that he would buy her a plane ticket at any time if she wanted to come for a visit. Eventually she agreed, and the door was opened to a great variety of values-consistent actions that were not previously possible. Most people would have fused with thoughts that a relationship was no longer possible, or even with thoughts that resulted in ineffective actions. But flexibility and a willingness to engage in actions that may fall short of what is ultimately desired can yield very tangible payoffs. More typically, this takes a less extreme form. For example, a man who values a loving, respectful, caring relationship with his wife might, in a moment of frustration, yell at her or be unfairly critical of her. The next moment is still an opportunity to act in a values-consistent manner. Commitment is essentially a moment-to-moment act.

The thought that you should or must commit to values-consistent behaviors can also become a trap. When a "should" or a "must" becomes verbally attached to an action, it can very quickly make that action aversive. As an example, I value being a loving, supportive, caring father who fully engages in the moment with my daughters, and I have had countless experiences when I have acted consistently with this value and found it very meaningful and vital. At times, however, after a long day at work, I have found myself fusing with thoughts that I "have to" act in this way, only to find that it seems like an unpleasant or difficult task. No one wants to be forced into an action, even if the action is one that previously seemed desirable. From a defusion perspective, however, "shoulds" and "musts" typically serve as markers for evaluative thoughts about "right" and "wrong." But such supposed obligations are not ironclad truths. What "must" be faced are the consequences of any given action, whether the action is consistent or inconsistent with a value. Ironically, when you have verbally freed yourself from any obligation to engage in valued living at a given moment, values-consistent action often becomes an even more attractive option.

While this issue will be addressed in greater detail in chapter 4, the moral relativity that defusion appears to introduce should be mentioned. If words are simply words and not a reflection of some ultimate universal Truth, it may seem that nothing is truly "right" or "wrong." In actuality, when defusion is anchored in direct experience in light of your values, a prosocial and moral sense of truth can emerge. In other words, if you are prompted to reflect on and trust your experiential sense of what feels meaningful, vital, and purposeful, that sense can come to serve as your moral compass. Of course, therapists using defusion techniques should be alert in case the client receives any kind of "anything goes" message, or uses defusion toward antisocial purposes.

Present-Moment Awareness and Defusion

Being fully in the present moment feels distinctly different than being absorbed in thought. There is a vivid, grounded sense of awareness involved in experiencing the present moment. By contrast, we have all frequently experienced riding trains of thought that have virtually nothing to do with what is happening to us presently, trains of thought that pull us completely away from sensing what is happening around us. Many times, our thoughts will begin as reflections on what we experience in a given moment. But even those thoughts, when fused with, immediately pull us out of the moment—a description or evaluation of something that just happened is, by definition, a description or evaluation of something that happened in the past. Thoughts and imagination can be vivid, but never as vivid as what is being seen, touched, tasted, felt, or heard here and now. This contrast between being in the present moment versus being caught in your head leads present-moment awareness to be a consistently available, effective defusion technique. When you have repeatedly experienced the sheer tangibility and vividness of the present-moment, in contrast to the relatively ethereal and insubstantial nature of thoughts, the notion that thoughts cannot capture the full breadth and depth of experience starts to ring true. This is the backbone of cognitive defusion. Repeatedly facilitating a sense of present moment awareness can do much to help build a context of defusion for a client, a context in which the client can begin to more consistently notice his problematic thoughts simply as thoughts.

Defusion and present-moment awareness share at least one other common feature. It is not uncommon to believe that contacting the present moment or defusing from our thoughts will reduce distress or result in a pleasant experience. Certainly, both processes can and often do provide some relief from distress. But they do not always appear to result in such relief, and believing thoughts that claim they do is bound to eventually result in failure. Great care is taken in ACT to get a client off the agenda of feeling better and thinking differently (along with all the associated and often counterproductive efforts) and onto an agenda of valued living and acceptance and defusion of difficult experiences that come with that living. Thus, an ACT client is oriented toward his direct experience of what works and what doesn't work when he slips back into using defusion and present-moment awareness primarily as tools to avoid distress. By definition, once this old goal is readopted, more time is spent avoiding and less time pursuing his values.

Self-as-Context and Defusion

A great deal of overlap exists between experiencing a sense of self-as-context and defusing from language. In fact, it seems as if the enactment of one process inexorably leads to the other. Simply noticing your thoughts as thoughts from an observer perspective typically leads to at least some degree of defusion. Defusing from a word or thought often results in noticing the formal or physical properties of words "out there" from an observer perspective. From a practitioner's standpoint, it is arguably not necessary to clearly distinguish between self-as-context and defusion techniques. However, techniques that put a primary and explicit focus on experiencing thoughts, feelings, and other sensations from an observer perspective typically fall into the self-as-context category. Defusion techniques, by contrast, primarily focus on breaking the rules of language.

Conclusion

Defusion is one of six core processes in ACT, along with self-as-context, acceptance, present-moment awareness, values, and a commitment to acting in accordance with those values. It is an indispensable part of ACT and interacts heavily with all of these processes in that context. Perhaps surprisingly, though, defusion can play an important role in other treatments as well. Rationales for using defusion in such treatments will be discussed at length in the next chapter.

CHAPTER 3

The Role of Defusion in Mindfulness-Based, Cognitive Behavioral, and Other Therapies

While "cognitive defusion" is a label that originated within ACT, many of the techniques and strategies subsumed under that label are not unique to ACT. Perhaps even more importantly, the psychological process referred to by defusion appears to be either already active in a variety of different treatments, or compatible with the theories underlying those treatments. This chapter will explore the broadly applicable nature of cognitive defusion—not only the critical role it can play in mindfulness-based treatments, but its compatibility with more broadly defined cognitive behavior therapies, as well as with treatments outside the CBT tradition.

Defusion and Mindfulness

The term "mindfulness," which originated within Buddhism, has been defined in various ways in the psychological literature. Each definition emphasizes some elements and attenuates or even eliminates others, which poses a difficulty in arriving at a universally agreed upon view of the concept. For example, Dimidjian and Linehan (2003) describe mindfulness as involving "the intentional process of observing, describing, and participating in reality nonjudgmentally, in the moment, and with effectiveness" (p. 229), while Kabat-Zinn (1994) defines it as "paying attention in a particular way: on purpose, in the present moment, and nonjudgmentally" (p. 4). Langer (2000) views mindfulness as a "flexible state of mind in which we are actively engaged in the present, noticing new things and sensitive to context…[as opposed to being] stuck in a single, rigid perspective…oblivious to alternative ways of knowing" (p. 220). Bishop and colleagues (2004) conceptualize mindfulness as "the self-regulation of attention so that it is maintained on immediate experience, thereby allowing for increased recognition of mental events in the present moment, [and] a particular orientation toward your experiences in the present moment, an orientation that is characterized by curiosity, openness, and acceptance" (p. 232).

Obvious commonalities exist between these definitions. An intentional focus on the present moment is clearly shared across all four, and an openness to or acceptance of present-moment experience is either explicitly mentioned or strongly implied. Attending to or observing aspects of your experience is also either explicitly mentioned or unavoidably implied in all four definitions as well. Something resembling defusion does not emerge as clearly from each of these sample conceptualizations, but is arguably either explicitly expressed or implied in them. The term "nonjudgmental" emerges in two definitions. While it is tempting to interpret "nonjudgmental" as an *absence* of judgment, the authors of those definitions offer further clarification. Dimidjian and Linehan (2003) add that mindfulness is "awareness simply of *what is*, at the level of *direct and immediate experience, separate from concepts, category, and expectations*" (p. 229; emphasis added). Similarly, Kabat-Zinn (1994) adds that "almost everything we see is labeled and categorized by the mind" (p. 33) and that we must "recognize this judging quality of mind…and intentionally assume the stance of an impartial witness by reminding [ourselves] to just observe it" (p. 34). Both clarifications indicate that mindfulness involves seeing and experiencing what is there to be experienced while at the same time not believing that the verbal judgments, categorizations, and labels our minds make adequately capture those experiences. This, in essence, is cognitive defusion.

Langer and Bishop do not explicitly allude to a clear defusion component to mindfulness in the quotations provided above, but further examination of their work strongly indicates that they, too, believe that some manner of not taking your thoughts too seriously is central to mindful action. Langer (2000) emphasizes the importance of viewing thoughts from diverse perspectives and realizing that they should be viewed in context and not taken as absolute truths, noting that while we are thinking, "all the while things are changing and at any one moment they are different from different perspectives, yet we hold them still in our minds as if they were constant" (p. 221). Langer's "flexible state of mind" thus refers to an explicit awareness that the "facts" presented to us by our thoughts should be viewed tentatively, as only "factual" to a degree. Bishop and colleagues (2004) clarify that mindfulness stands in contradiction to "getting caught up in ruminative, elaborative, thought streams *about* your experience," and instead "involves a direct *experience* of events" (p. 232), a clarification that clearly invokes defusion.

This sampling of scientific definitions for mindfulness outside the confines of acceptance and commitment therapy seem to converge on the importance of some version of "not taking your thoughts too seriously" or as substitutes for direct experience. Within ACT, defusion has been viewed as a process integral to mindfulness for some time. Fletcher and Hayes (2005) stated that mindfulness might be usefully construed as a combination of present-moment awareness, a sense of self-as-context, an open and accepting stance toward your experience, and a defused perspective toward your thoughts. Defusion, from their perspective, facilitates the accepting, present-moment awareness inherent in mindfulness because it "undermines the excessive [often negative] literal impact of language" to make experience more acceptable, and because it undermines "temporal and evaluative [language] that move[s] the focus away from 'now'" (p. 322). In other words, defusion makes it less difficult to accept our experience because it disrupts our negative verbal evaluations of that experience, and hinders language's ability to carry us away from the present moment to musings about the past and the future. Defusion is an integral part of mindfulness.

Enhancing Mindfulness-Based Therapies with Defusion Techniques

Many different empirically supported mindfulness-based treatments are currently in use. Mindfulness-based stress reduction (MBSR) has been used to effectively treat psychological distress associated with chronic pain (Kabat-Zinn, 1982), anxiety disorders (Kabat-Zinn et al., 1992), and cancer (Massion, Teas, Hebert, Wertheimer, & Kabat-Zinn, 1995), among other problems. Mindfulness-based cognitive therapy (MBCT; Segal, Williams, & Teasdale, 2002) has considerable evidence supporting its effectiveness in treating depression (McCarney, Schulz, & Grey, 2012). Dialectical behavior therapy (DBT; see, for example, Linehan, 1993), which relies on mindfulness exercises as a strong treatment component, has been repeatedly found effective in treating symptoms of borderline personality disorder (Kliem, Kröger, & Kosfelder, 2010). A recent meta-analysis including 209 published empirical outcome studies indicated that mindfulness-based treatments in general were effective in treating a variety of psychological disorders, and as effective as cognitive behavior therapy and pharmacological treatments in the nine studies in which they were compared (Khoury et al., 2013).

These treatments largely rely on some kind of formal sitting meditation; mindfulness activities, such as mindfulness of physical sensations while walking, exercising, showering, driving, doing dishes, and so on (see, for example, Spradlin, 2002, pp. 57–61); or mindfulness of the physical and cognitive aspects of emotions (see, for example, Spradlin, 2002, pp. 62–65) to help clients respond to thoughts, feelings, and other aspects of their experience in a flexible, adaptive, and effective manner. Considering that these have historically been the techniques used to promote mindfulness (in Buddhism, for example), this should come as no surprise. But if defusion is accurately understood as being an important component of mindfulness, and if we bear in mind the positive effects of existing defusion studies discussed in chapter 10, utilizing additional defusion strategies in such treatments would expand the range of techniques available. Considering that some techniques work for some people but not for others, and that there can be significant barriers to regularly engaging in formal sitting meditation (Williams, Van Ness, Jane, & McCorkle, 2012), the kinds of defusion techniques discussed in this book might be a welcome addition to many forms of mindfulness therapy.

In fact, some techniques that do not resemble formal meditation or simple mindful awareness of experience but do resemble common ACT defusion techniques are already in documented use in some mindfulness-based therapies. In many cases, of course, these commonalities likely reflect the common mindfulness-based lineage of these treatments, and do not imply that ACT practitioners or theorists "invented" the techniques. For example, Linehan (1993) has noted that teaching "'what' skills" (pp. 63–67), in which clients are explicitly encouraged to find words that simply describe their moment-to-moment experiences and to be wary of and "unglue" (p. 121) themselves from opinion words that evaluate that experience, is a standard part of DBT. This strategy bears some resemblance to the description-evaluation defusion exercise detailed in chapter 7 of this book, a common ACT defusion exercise first described by Hayes et al. (1999). Segal and colleagues (2002) described an MBCT metaphor (among several metaphors comparable to ACT defusion and self-as-context techniques) that compares recurrent problematic thoughts to a "tape in the mind" (pp. 252–255) that repeatedly plays back under certain circumstances, so as to highlight the insidious yet ultimately suspicious nature of thoughts. The metaphor resembles both the computer programming and "bad news radio" defusion metaphors used in ACT (see, for example, Hayes & Smith, 2005). MBCT practitioners are also directed to promote an understanding of the distinction between "facts" and "interpretations" (Segal et al., 2002, pp. 254–257) that is markedly similar to the distinction made between descriptions and evaluations in ACT. Furthermore, mindfulness-based relapse prevention (MBRP) therapists have been advised, for example, to help their clients to metaphorically liken their thoughts to "images or words on a movie screen or balloons floating away," or "a radio broadcast or to a tiny creature on your shoulder delivering a running commentary" (Bowen, Chawla, & Marlatt, 2010, p. 131). Such strategies closely resemble common ACT defusion and self-as-context techniques, but differ in form from the types of traditional Buddhist meditation and mindfulness practices that dominate most mindfulness-based treatments. If finding a more flexible and varied array of mindfulness strategies within these treatments is deemed desirable and potentially useful, then incorporating a range of ACT-based defusion techniques becomes an attractive option.

Integrating Defusion Techniques into Conventional Cognitive Behavior Therapy

Defusion and cognitive restructuring appear to be very much at odds: the latter assumes that thoughts must change for behavior to change, while the former assumes that thought change doesn't matter. At first glance, it would appear that cognitive behavior therapy is out of necessity based on a cognitive model similar to that advocated by Beck (1976), in which thoughts cause problematic behaviors and emotions and must be changed before those behaviors and emotions can change. Hofmann, Asmundson, and Beck (2013) hold this view, and recently emphasized that, in cognitive behavior therapy, "negative emotions and harmful behaviors are products of dysfunctional thoughts and cognitive distortions" (p. 6). If this were a binding assumption held by all cognitive behavior therapists, then it would mandate the use of cognitive restructuring and contraindicate the use of defusion in CBT, since defusion techniques are grounded in the assumption that thoughts do *not* have to change in order for emotional and overt behavioral change to occur.

However, others have argued that the type of CBT described by Hofmann and colleagues (2013) is more properly labeled "cognitive therapy." Herbert and Forman (2013) argued that the term "cognitive behavior therapy" "does not describe a particular theory, psychotherapy model, or group of technologies, but rather a very broad family of psychotherapies that share core cognitive and behavioral strategies as well as a commitment to scientific empiricism" (p. 219). While Beck's (1976) signature cognitive version of CBT adopts an exclusive cognitive model and necessitates the use of cognitive restructuring, other forms of CBT, such as ACT, DBT, and MBCT, address problematic cognitions in different ways, and represent variations in opinion about how cognition interacts with behavior and emotions. Dobson and Dozois (2010, p. 4) offer the perspective that the assumptions that unite the different varieties of CBT are:

1. Cognitive activity affects behavior.

2. Cognitive activity may be monitored or altered.

3. Desired behavior change *may* [emphasis added] be affected through cognitive change.

Viewed from these perspectives, CBT in the broader sense appears to allow for a variety of ways of addressing problematic cognitions, with defusion or other cognitive strategies being potentially as viable as restructuring techniques.

In fact, Dobson (2013) has argued that the field of CBT is actually moving "toward a metacognitive model of change" (p. 224). Metacognition refers to thoughts you have about other thoughts or about other aspects of your experience. CBT treatments that pay explicit attention to metacognition typically do not rely on cognitive restructuring as an exclusive or primary change strategy, nor do they dispense with it altogether. In metacognitive therapy (Wells, 2008), much of the focus is on relating to problematic thoughts in different ways and learning to direct attention away from dysfunctional ruminative thoughts and toward more useful information. Typically, the only thoughts that are cognitively challenged are those that involve clients' beliefs that they must continue their ruminative cycle. In MBCT, clients are prompted to become more aware of their thoughts (and other experiences), not in an effort to change them, but rather to learn how to "sit with" them without becoming reactive (Segal et al., 2002). In DBT, clients are taught to evaluate problematic thoughts and urges from a "wise mind" perspective, and such thoughts are experienced from a mindful perspective with an understanding that they do not have to be changed (Linehan, 1993). And in ACT, of course, noticing your thoughts (and thoughts about thoughts) and learning to relate to all of them differently is ubiquitous. Whether or not CBT will continue moving in a metacognitive direction, such observations illustrate that there are a variety of ways of addressing problematic thoughts and of viewing the causality or noncausality of cognition in CBT.

Mixed Messages: Combining Defusion and Cognitive Restructuring

While it has hopefully been established that using cognitive strategies other than restructuring in CBT is fair game, and that thoughts do not *have* to cause behavior, a potential problem arises when using defusion and restructuring in tandem. Defusion essentially teaches that thoughts do not have to change in order for overt behavior to change, that the war of words need not be won before emotions can be accepted for what they are. The use of restructuring techniques implies that difficult thoughts can and must be changed in order to move forward. Additionally, if a therapist—and by extension, the client—is not explicitly clear that defusion and restructuring are simply two different ways of changing behavior *and* that you can behave in a way that is inconsistent with your thoughts, confusion and diluted treatment effects may result.

It should be made clear that there is currently no data exploring the effects of mixing defusion and restructuring techniques—or mixing an attenuated version of the cognitive model with an assumption that thoughts do not cause behavior—in therapy. While there is data that indicates that mindfulness-based therapy (specifically, MBCT) reduces relapse in clients who had previously received cognitive therapy for depression (Segal et al., 2002), no currently published studies have formally evaluated a mixture of defusion and restructuring. If they were combined, the most sensible approach would likely involve starting with the explicit shared assumptions that (1) thoughts rarely, if ever, capture the full breadth and depth of the experiences or facts they claim to describe; (2) compelling thoughts influence our emotions and behaviors, but they do not force us to act or feel in ways that are consistent with them; and (3) defusion and restructuring strategies are simply different tools that can be used to change behavior when problematic thoughts and feelings arise. In other words, it may be helpful to change the way you think when possible, while at the same time reminding yourself, through the use of defusion strategies, that it is not necessary to change thoughts because they do not capture absolute truth anyway. If a given client gravitates toward restructuring techniques and finds them successful in changing many of his cognitions, then well and good. Defusion strategies could be used when restructuring fails, or could be used as a frontline approach by clients who embrace their message. Empirically, it may turn out that clients with a relative deficit in logical, rational thinking may benefit from using restructuring techniques as a frontline strategy, while clients with no such deficit may benefit from using defusion. Additionally, it may prove that clients facing great or chronic distress and who view their situations with relative realism are better served by defusion strategies, while those in other situations make more effective use of restructuring.

Using Defusion in Other Forms of Therapy

The fundamental message behind defusion is that words do not capture absolute truth, and that the words that increase our suffering are therefore not binding. From this perspective, it would seem that any brand of psychotherapy that implicitly or explicitly acknowledges that our thoughts and impressions contribute to our problems might be able to make use of defusion strategies. Defusion is of more obvious relevance to certain types of therapy. Constructivist treatments, for example, actively target the role we play in constructing the narratives of ourselves and the world around us, seeking to deconstruct problematic narratives and build more adaptive ones. Defusion could be of great help in deconstructing an old narrative, and could also make new narratives more flexible and continually adaptive. Other, more "postmodern" approaches to therapy could also benefit from the use of defusion strategies, since such strategies may, for example, help weaken the hold of prescribed yet problematic ways of thinking. Existential therapists have acknowledged the vital importance of a struggle for meaning in a world where meaning is not etched in stone. Defusion strategies might, for example, help an existential therapy client realize that even the thought, "Life has no meaning," is suspect, and that meaning arises in the vitality of living and embracing life.

Defusion could play a role even in treatments where the notion that words are misleading does not take center stage. A psychodynamic therapist working toward her client's emotional insight could use defusion to help the client unhook from troublesome interpersonal appraisals learned in past relationships and problematically applied in current ones. A humanistic therapist helping a client see and accept himself as he is could use defusion to cut through his negative self-evaluations and thoughts about who he should or must be. And a gestalt therapist could use defusion to help a client become more reliant on her direct experiences and less reliant on verbal interpretations, especially those interpretations that cause problems.

The rationale and caveats for using defusion techniques in conventional cognitive behavior therapy apply to other forms of therapy as well. Therapists who adopt a position that thoughts cause behavior and must be changed for psychological progress to occur will likely send counterproductive mixed messages to clients if they use defusion techniques. Therapists who assume that thoughts do not need to change prior to behavior change, who make this assumption consistently clear to the client, and who do not use other techniques in a way that implies that thought change is a necessity may well be able to successfully integrate defusion into their practice.

Conclusion

I have argued that defusion can be used in a wide variety of psychotherapeutic treatments. While its applicability to mindfulness-based treatments, for example, may be obvious because of ACT's continuation of the mindfulness tradition, defusion may even be a viable tool for use in more conventional forms of CBT—treatments often seen as mandating cognitive change. With the caveats discussed in this chapter, defusion may prove to be a welcome adjunct to any treatment that does not explicitly endorse the belief that thoughts must change for behavior and emotions to change.

CHAPTER 4

Laying the Foundation
for Defusion

The next five chapters will explain how to introduce defusion strategies to clients, and how to implement a variety of different techniques that use defusion. Before using many of the more explicit defusion techniques, however, a number of factors need to be considered. First, since some defusion techniques may seem rather odd to clients, I will provide some tips for introducing defusion in a relatively natural manner. Next, I will focus on the importance of seeding in sufficient therapist empathy to minimize defusion's potential for making clients feel invalidated. Then I will consider issues that may arise when mixing defusion and cognitive restructuring techniques. Finally, I will underscore the importance of tempering defusion with an existential sense of meaning and morality.

The Oddness of Defusion

As you may have noticed in chapter 1, some defusion techniques are, quite frankly, weird. Much of this is by design. To break the rules of "language as usual," which are so ubiquitous and entrenched that they are typically not even noticed, some pretty odd or unexpected things need to happen. While this oddness can be effective, it can also be off-putting if not offered in the proper context. Imagine, for example, asking a distressed client within the first ten minutes of the first session to repeat the word "milk" over and over, without providing a rationale for the exercise and without having yet developed a trusting therapeutic relationship. Such an intervention might be well received, but there is likely a greater chance that the client would not return for a second session.

A number of more subtle defusion techniques (such as the "mind" and "thought" methods presented in detail in chapter 5) can be easily seeded into conversation within minutes of the first therapeutic contact. But the more invasive defusion techniques may require at least a brief but explicit nod to the rationale behind defusion—the fact that language is suspect, that words often do not accurately correspond to the full depth and breadth of "reality." Chapter 5 provides several examples of what such a rationale might look like, as well as some ways you can introduce defusion techniques that do not immediately appear relevant to what the client is disclosing. A good rule of thumb might involve gauging your own reactions to each defusion technique presented in this book. If you are relatively new to defusion and perceive a technique as weird, or not immediately therapeutically relevant, chances may be good that your clients will perceive it that way as well. You should bear in mind, however, that your client may see a technique as weird even if you do not. Once the premise of defusion is made clear to a client, the need to introduce rationales for subsequent defusion techniques fades away.

Defusion and Invalidation

Defusion strategies run the risk of invalidating a client's subjective experience. At its core, defusion means that the stories we tell about our lives and our struggles are not absolute truths. But if defusion work is not conducted in proper fashion, it can be easy for a client to miss the global nature of this assertion and to believe the therapist thinks the client's particular story is not true. Giving a client the impression that you doubt her ability to correctly identify the facts in a life that she has lived a long time and that you are just getting familiar with typically does not bode well. Defusion techniques can also seem to trivialize a client's distress if used in a cavalier fashion. Imagine asking a client, in the first session, to sing his most distressing thoughts to the tune of his favorite pop song. A deep sense of invalidation might well result. The effectiveness and appropriateness of more invasive defusion techniques depend on a good therapeutic relationship in which the client knows that the therapist empathizes very well with him. Furthermore, the client should know the rationale behind the use of such techniques, and should understand that the misleading character of words and thoughts is not a personal shortcoming, but something we all grapple with.

Mixing Defusion and Thought Change Strategies

Guidelines for integrating defusion strategies with cognitive restructuring within the context of CBT were offered in chapter 3. It should be noted that these guidelines may need to be put into action when defusion is used in other forms of treatment as well. Attempting to change the way another person thinks about his experiences tends to be a default mode for human beings. We are all taught from a young age to try to think about things accurately and rationally, and this sensibility may seep into our therapeutic work even when we use a theoretical approach to treatment that does not explicitly aim at thought change. One example of this tendency might occur when we encourage a client to "make sense" of what has happened to her in a way that either provides comfort or that "allows" her to move forward in a relatively constructive manner. While it is certainly nice to find an "accurate" and relatively constructive way of thinking about your difficulties, it might be counterproductive to send the message that you *must* arrive at such a way of thinking to move forward. From a defusion perspective, thoughts do not have to change in order for constructive movement to be made. They simply need to be held lightly.

A similar example might involve clients believing they must have insight into exactly why they have their current psychological problems before they can rise above them. While knowing some causes of our problems can be beneficial (for example, when an ongoing contributor to distress and disability can be identified and changed), often the perceived causes are rather distant and immutable. We generally believe we must have thoughts that accurately capture the reality of what caused our current situation. Yet from a defusion perspective, many of these thoughts are simply part of a semifictional narrative—a narrative which may make sense, but which is not necessary for moving forward through our current problems. Regardless of which variation of the need and the effort to have the "right thoughts" arises in therapy, the "necessity" of those "needs" should be explicitly held lightly by both therapist and client if defusion strategies are in use. Otherwise, the central message defusion is intended to convey—that the problematic and distressing thoughts we struggle with are not absolute truths and do not need to change—can be undermined.

Defusion and Meaninglessness: Grounding Defusion in Values

When defusion is taken to its logical extreme, a sort of existential crisis can result. If our thoughts are not absolute truths, then it may seem that there is no absolute meaning, no right or wrong, and perhaps even no absolute point of reference. Although I have encountered this extreme conclusion in only a few of my clients, the potential clearly exists. In ACT, this potential meaninglessness and amorality is counterbalanced by elaborating on the clients' direct experience of what matters most to them—on their own deeply held personal values. In other words, clients are asked to get clear about specific ways of living, treating others, and engaging with various domains of their lives that give them an increased sense of vitality, meaning, and purpose. Inevitably, these values are at least a partial product of experiences they have had firsthand, whether they have been on the giving or receiving end of the values they endorse. These direct experiences are then used to trump thoughts that doubt whether they *really* value those ways of living or whether their values *really* matter. A client might say something like, "I want to be kind to other people—I want to treat them fairly and compassionately, to connect with them as human beings." Subsequently, the client might start to doubt whether this value *really* matters to him and might even doubt whether treating others this way ultimately even matters. After all, the values statement is simply made up of words, and words do not appear to capture absolute truth. In such a case, the therapist can evoke a different kind of knowing—the kind of direct experiential knowing that we have when doing things a particular way simply feels right and vital, and matters greatly at a personal level. An exchange between therapist and client like this might go as follows:

Client: I don't know. My mind *says* it's important to treat people this way, that it really matters. But what's the point? They're all just words, evaluations at that, and I've been noticing a lot lately how flimsy those kinds of words are. It looks like, ultimately, it just doesn't matter.

Therapist: So you're having a thought, "Ultimately, it just doesn't matter." It also seems like you're having a thought like, "Because it ultimately doesn't matter, that negates my value of connecting with other people, with treating them compassionately and kindly." Am I right on that?

Client: Yeah, that's it. Sometimes it feels like it really matters, but then I realize it doesn't.

Therapist: Let me ask you something. I remember you telling me about a really good, heartfelt interaction you had with Carl, that administrative assistant where you work, somebody who gets overlooked and kind of treated one-dimensionally. Can you tell me what that felt like again?

Client: It felt really good. He's a really nice guy, and it seemed to mean a lot to him that a coworker really took the time to get to know him and didn't just put one more job on his plate. It meant something to me, too—it made my day better to have a genuine, caring interaction like that.

Therapist: So it sounds like your direct experience is telling you that it mattered a lot to you—and to him, too, for that matter—to treat him that way. You were doing something that's important to you, something that just feels right to you. And when you think back to other times you've really connected with others, what was your direct experience then?

Client: Pretty much the same. It almost always feels good. It's important to me.

Therapist: And notice how your mind has been trying to convince you that it's somehow not "etched in stone" somewhere in the universe that it absolutely, truly matters to connect with others. That, because of that thought, it doesn't matter at all. And what if that is all just talk, too? What's more important, and what feels more concrete, more tangible—what your mind says, or what you actually experience when you connect with others?

Client: Well, those connections feel real. The good feelings that come out of them are real.

Therapist: So it feels like connecting with others really does matter to *you*, that it's worth doing, that it makes life better?

Client: Yes, definitely.

Therapist: If that's the case, does it matter what your mind says?

Client: [*Laughing.*] I guess not!

Embedded throughout this dialogue are not only explicit references to a core client value and contrasts between the client's mind and his direct experience, but also defusion prompts leveled at thoughts that doubt the absolute importance of his interpersonal connection value. Thoughts that doubt the veracity of thoughts in general are useful so long as they are helpful, but they, too, are just thoughts and can be treated as such if they start to contribute to the kind of existential meaninglessness our fictional client was starting to demonstrate. More generally, the lessons defusion teaches can logically result in a thought like, "Words cannot capture reality," but that, too, is just a thought. We ultimately do not know if *that* thought is true. Fortunately, defusion also teaches that we do not have to change that thought to get on with our lives, to trust our direct experiences about what matters to us and move in those directions. Any thoughts, held lightly, can be carried on that journey.

The same holds true for thoughts about how ethical behavior does not matter because there is no fixed, immutable ethical code sewn into the fabric of the universe. While I have never had an ACT client who genuinely, after careful reflection, endorsed an antisocial or amoral value, the possibility exists that some clients might use defusion to justify antisocial or destructively amoral behavior. Drilling down to key client experiences about what it felt like to help and connect with others, in contrast to what it felt like to engage in various amoral or antisocial behaviors, can be instrumental in helping clients realize that specific prosocial, constructive ways of living really do matter to them, regardless of an apparent lack of explicit endorsement by the universe.

Existentialists have grappled with this aspect of humanity for centuries, and the fundamental issue focused on has likely been around almost as long as humans have used language. In the face of a vast and virtually incomprehensible universe, human beings are confronted with the thought that nothing matters in and of itself, that the universe does not come with an *a priori* declaration of what matters and what is worth striving for, and that we must make our own meanings and forge our own ethical codes. Once you realize that your mind is not your most trustworthy friend, you must ultimately rely on your experiences to tell you what matters, what is meaningful and important to *you*. Words can be helpful or unhelpful in assisting those realizations, but they should not be allowed to negate them.

Conclusion

In summary, even though a number of defusion techniques can be odd and potentially off-putting, they can be seamlessly introduced in a variety of ways (chapter 5 will provide many additional examples). A high degree of therapist empathy is critically important when using defusion, given the process's potential to invalidate the client's experience. Careful considerations of how to use both defusion and cognitive restructuring techniques with the same client should be made to help prevent the messages of both sets of techniques from becoming muddled. And finally, effort may be needed to counter a sense of existential meaninglessness if the client concludes that nothing has meaning because words have no meaning.

The following five chapters explain how to introduce and use a variety of different defusion techniques. Chapter 5 contains many examples of how to introduce defusion early in treatment, while chapters 6 through 9 discuss different categories of defusion techniques. It is important to remember that flexibility is key when using defusion, or virtually any therapeutic technique. While these techniques are discussed in very specific ways here, especially in the fictional therapy transcripts that illustrate their uses, there are numerous other ways these techniques could be used. Feel free to adapt them so that they better suit your personal style and your client's needs.

CHAPTER 5

Introducing Defusion in Treatment

The phenomenon referred to as defusion runs counter to a lifetime of learning, where words are believed to capture our experiences with relative accuracy and where the best words capture absolute truth. Given that therapist and client alike share this history with words, and given the initial oddity of many defusion techniques, therapists new to defusion often have difficulty introducing defusion techniques seamlessly and effectively. Fortunately, there are many ways to accomplish this, several of which will be discussed in this chapter. Note that the word "defusion" is rarely ever introduced to clients, and technical descriptions of it are even more rarely discussed in therapy. Rather, effective attempts to instantiate defusion in a therapy session simply help identify thoughts as thoughts, and highlight, *in vivo*, how inadequate these thoughts are at capturing the full truth of direct experience.

Using "Mind" and "Thought" Language Conventions

Less invasive defusion techniques, such as those that subtly identify thoughts as thoughts or as products of the mind, can be seeded in as early as an intake session. While the effects of using such language conventions are typically not dramatic, they can often generate a bit of distance between clients and their thoughts, and help lay a foundation for more intensive defusion work. Their use is demonstrated in the following short dialogue.

Client: For the longest time, I've felt like I'm just different, like I just don't belong.

Therapist: So you've had this thought, "I just don't belong," for a long time. What other thoughts show up when you think you don't belong?

Client: Well, I'm not interested in the things that my friends are interested in. I feel out of sync with them. Sometimes I worry there's just something wrong with me.

Therapist: Ouch—that would be a tough thought to have: "There's something wrong with me." Can I ask, when that thought comes up, what other thoughts show up?

Client: Just that, well, I feel really disconnected from people. I think it's because I'm really awkward, I don't know how to talk to people very well. I just feel like I'm an idiot sometimes.

Therapist: Yeah, those are some more tough thoughts to have: "I'm an idiot," "I'm really awkward." As you think those thoughts, what feelings show up?

Client: I actually feel kind of bad. Sad, really. Kind of ashamed.

Therapist: [Leans forward, nods empathically.] Yeah. Even just talking about it makes those feelings come up. [Pauses.] Are there other thoughts running through your mind right now?

Several aspects of this dialogue should be noted. First, it is hopefully apparent that the subtle defusion work demonstrated could occur alongside a number of other therapeutic agendas, including assessment and rapport-building. These "thought" and "mind" language conventions can be used with greater or lesser consistency, though less use would do less to help build a context of defusion within treatment that allows the client to more consistently see her thoughts simply as thoughts. Second, note how not all thoughts were labeled as such by the therapist. Problematic, evaluative thoughts were the prime candidates. The goal is not to get the client to defuse from all thoughts, but from those that cause problems when taken literally (though it is desirable to build a client's general ability to "hold thoughts lightly," or not take any thoughts *too* seriously). Third, the therapist should consistently express empathy for the distress the client is experiencing, as simply labeling one thought after another as a thought might seem invalidating. Finally, it should be noted that there typically isn't a sense of "mission accomplished" on the therapist's part when simply using "thought" and "mind" language conventions in the way they are implemented in this dialogue. In other words, while such use can create some distance between a client and her thoughts and help her more readily experience emotions attached to them, it usually does not result in an explicit client awareness that thoughts are just nonbinding verbal utterances. Other defusion techniques can be folded in later to build on this experience.

Client-Initiated Defusion

Perhaps the best way to introduce defusion is in response to a natural skepticism the client expresses toward one of her own thoughts, whether in the past or in the present. For example, after a few sessions, one client with pervasive anger issues remarked that he used to get extremely angry at his wife when he could not locate one of his possessions in the house, under the assumption that she had moved it without his knowledge. After yelling at and criticizing her repeatedly, only to find later that he himself had misplaced the possession, he started to realize that he could not trust his suspicions in such situations. The exchange went something like this:

> *Therapist:* And so, when you reflected on the past and realized you couldn't trust your mind when something of yours went missing at home, did it lessen the anger or make the suspicions any weaker?
>
> *Client:* No. I had to work really hard. I still get really angry and immediately suspect my wife, but I've learned not to follow

through on that. I guess you could say I don't act out on my anger.

Therapist: Hmm. [*Nods appreciatively.*] And before learning that your thoughts in those situations were suspect, how convinced were you that she had moved your stuff?

Client: Completely convinced. Not a doubt in my mind.

Therapist: I've noticed my mind do the same thing—be convinced that all the thoughts I'm having are true, only to find out later that, wait a minute, they were off. Are there other times when you've noticed that—when you've noticed that you were convinced about something and later learned it just wasn't so?

Client: [*Pauses.*] Yeah, yeah, that happens sometimes. [*Client mentions a couple of other instances when this has occurred.*]

Therapist: Well, here's the thing. Minds are pretty good at convincing us of things, especially when strong emotions are there. Like, when we're really anxious, minds are pretty good at convincing us that our worst fears are going to come true. When we're really angry, minds are pretty good at convincing us that our wives did something wrong.

Client: You got that right.

Therapist: I wonder if that happens a lot more often than we realize. I mean, what if we get so used to trusting what our minds say—because they're very convincing and shout pretty loud at us—that we take most of our thoughts for granted, even when they don't correspond completely to reality? I mean, what if our minds are taking us for a ride more often than we realize?

Client: [*Pauses.*] I guess…I mean, I guess they could.

Therapist: And I wonder….You've described a number of situations in the past few weeks where you've gotten angry, and in some cases acted on that anger in a way that got you in trouble—got you fired from jobs, led to difficulties with the police. And I guess I kind of want to ask permission. You've had the experience of getting angry with your wife and noticing that your mind wasn't telling the complete truth in those situations. You've had the experience that your mind has led you astray in other areas of your life. In coming sessions, would you be willing to look at some of the thoughts that show up when you get angry, in other situations, from this perspective—from this perspective of being suspicious about how absolutely true all of those thoughts are?

Client: We could try.

This is just one example of how an opportunity for defusion can be naturally initiated by a client. A similar exchange could readily be prompted by asking a client if he can recall a time when he believed something very strongly and then realized his belief was not true. The exchange above also illustrates the importance of surrounding defusion-based prompts with empathy and validation, especially at first. The therapist openly admits that his mind does things very similar to the client's, thereby hinting that perhaps both therapist and client get fooled by their minds more often than they know, in an attempt to validate the client and avoid defensiveness. Similarly, the therapist asks for permission to view additional client experiences from a defusion-based perspective—a permission that is extremely important with clients who hold their thoughts very rigidly and defensively.

Looking at Thoughts Versus Looking Through Thoughts

Chris McCurry, a clinical psychologist and author with nearly twenty years of ACT experience with children and adolescents, often uses a variant of the Hayes and colleagues (1999; 2012) "looking at versus looking through" technique to provide a very concrete way of introducing defusion. Its concreteness is not only arguably necessary to explain an abstract concept to young, developing minds, but may well facilitate its introduction to adults as well. The exercise utilizes physical props—in this case, a pair of safety goggles with yellow lenses, or a pair of "bug eye" goggles that produce multiple copies of whatever is being viewed. The following dialogue (adapted with permission from Dr. McCurry) illustrates their use, after the client is asked to put the goggles on.

> *Therapist:* Now, what color is the room? [*Or in the case of the bug eyes,* "How many of me do you see now?"]

> *Client:* It's yellow. [*Or,* "There are four of you."]

> *Therapist:* Is it really yellow all of a sudden?

> *Client:* No, it's because of these. [*Taps the lenses.*]

> *Therapist:* Right, the glasses make the room look yellow.

> [*At this point, therapist and client discuss whatever type of psychological goggles cause problems for the client—anxiety goggles, anger goggles, "I can't do math" goggles, and so on. Both therapist and client hold a pair of goggles.*]

> *Therapist:* Imagine that these were "anxiety goggles." Whenever you wear them [*puts them in front of eyes*], they make everything look scary, just like these goggles make everything look yellow. But what if you take them off? [*Holds goggles to the side.*] The anxiety hasn't gone anywhere. It's still here [*points to goggles*] saying, "The world is scary. I'm too anxious to do it." But now I can see so much else and can keep this thought from making my decisions for me as if it were real and true. Does that make sense?

> *Client:* [*Puts goggles in front of his eyes, then moves them to the side.*] Yes, it's like when you think there's a monster in the room and you get scared, but then you remember there are no monsters. You think you see him when the goggles are on, but you see that he might not be there when you take them off. It's still scary, though.

Therapist: Yes. You're scared, but you realize that fear doesn't have to push you around—that even though you're scared, it doesn't mean something really, really bad has to happen. And sometimes your goggles are stuck on pretty tight. But you can remind yourself it's just those goggles again making things appear a certain way. Then you can slow down and think about your next move.

The Description-Evaluation Technique

A variant of the "bad cup" metaphor developed by Hayes and colleagues (1999; 2012), the description-evaluation technique is used to help distinguish between physically descriptive language that points to the client's direct experience, and evaluative language that pretends to derive absolute truths about the implications of the experiences. It is all too easy for our minds to negatively evaluate the world, others, and our own actions, experiences, character, potential, and so on in ways that are unnecessarily convincing and problematic. This technique can help the client see the contrast between the solidity of direct experience pointed to by descriptive language and the ethereality (as in lack of material substance) of indirect or evaluative language. It can also introduce the core message of defusion in a clear, systematic, and fluid manner. If the client finds the distinction between descriptions and evaluations helpful, the therapist can build on the experience in later sessions by strategically asking the client to identify which labels apply to currently experienced problematic thoughts. It should be noted that the distinction between descriptions and evaluations is first applied, below, to an emotionally neutral object, and is then later applied to the issue that is distressing the client. This is because noticing that distinction can be difficult when it is first applied to difficult thoughts and emotions. Experiencing the distinction first with a neutral object is intended to boost the client's ability to spot it even when difficult thoughts and feelings might interfere.

Client: It's just, I'm not good with people. I want to have friends, but I get so anxious. There's just something wrong with me.

Therapist: And that thought, "There's just something wrong with me"—what other thoughts show up along with that?

Client: I don't know. I guess, I just say dumb things. I'm not interesting. I feel like I'm not worth getting to know. Man, I feel depressed, anxious just thinking about it.

Therapist: That's a lot to carry—that anxiety, that sadness…those tough thoughts. And I know you've felt trapped by all this for a long time, haven't you?

Client: Yeah.

Therapist: Sometimes with thoughts and feelings this tough, it can help to look at them from a little bit different angle. To pull those thoughts apart and see what's underneath them. Would you be willing to give that a try?

Client: I guess so. What do you have in mind?

Therapist: Well, there are two different kinds of thoughts that we have, and when we mistake one kind for another, it can cause problems. I'd like to make a distinction between those two different kinds of thoughts—descriptions and evaluations—and apply this distinction to the thoughts you've been struggling with. I'd like to make the distinction first with something pretty basic so I can make sure I'm explaining it clearly—and then once it's clear, we'll look at your thoughts from the same perspective. Would that be okay—if we have a brief diversion, and then use that to take a new look at those old thoughts?

Client: Okay.

Therapist: Great. There are two types of thoughts—descriptions and evaluations. Descriptive thoughts point out any aspect of something that you can perceive with one of your five senses. So if you can see it, smell it, touch it, taste it, or hear it, it's a description. Anything else you can say about something or someone is an evaluation. With that in mind, could you give me some descriptions of this table? [*Pats hand on table.*]

Client: Well, it's made out of wood.

Therapist: Yeah, definitely—you can see that clearly with your eyes. What else?

Client: It's solid.

Therapist: Yes. [*Pounds table with hand.*] Yeah, you can feel how solid it is. What else?

Client: It's brown. It's shaped like a rectangle.

Therapist: Good, all things that you can see. And it has four legs—they look like some kind of metal. It's got black plastic on the edges. All descriptions? All things that you can directly see?

Client: Yes.

Therapist: And this may sound like an odd question now, but hopefully it will make more sense in a little bit. The "wood-ness," the "solidness," the "rectangular-ness" of this table—are those part of the table just as it is, or are they something that our minds add to the table?

Client: Uh, I don't think I get it.

Therapist: Would the wood, the solidness, the rectangular shape still be here even if we weren't here to label it that way? Are they simply part of the table?

Client: Yes, definitely.

Therapist: Okay. Now let's find some evaluations of this table. Remember, I told you evaluations are any way that you can talk about the table that isn't just a simple description of its physical features. Can you evaluate this table for me?

Client: Well, it's a nice table.

Therapist: Okay, good. It's pretty. What else?

Client: It looks useful.

Therapist: Good. And do you think somebody could come in and say, "It's an ugly table," or "It's useless," or "It's a piece of junk," or "It's the best table ever"?

Client: [*Laughs.*] Yeah, I suppose somebody could. It's like there's a kind of subjective quality to it.

Therapist: Yes, there is, isn't there? Now let me ask you this. The "niceness," the "ugliness," the "usefulness," the "uselessness"—are those simply part of the table, or are they something that our minds add to the table?

Client: I guess they are something our minds add to the table.

Therapist: And "nice," "ugly," "useful," "useless"—are they as solid as "wood" or "hard"? [*Bangs on table.*] Can you grab them [*extends grasping hand out into thin air as if trying to grab on to a thought*] in the same way that you can grab this table? [*Grabs table.*] Isn't there something kind of airy, kind of fishy about those evaluations?

Client: Yeah, it's like they pretend to be right, but when you look closer they are just kind of subjective.

On many occasions throughout this dialogue, the therapist pats or pounds on the table and asks questions like, "Can you grab this [*specific evaluation*] in the same way you can grab this table?" This is done to emphasize the perceptual solidity that descriptive language refers to, to try to help create an experience of certainty that what is being described is really there and to help contrast that perceptual solidity with the relative "airiness" of evaluative language. Evaluations simply cannot be firmly grasped (or seen, or tasted) like objects described can—and if they are not objectively "solid," how much can they be trusted? To help sharpen this distinction, it is advisable to pick an object with some very robust physical characteristics. I prefer using a table or desk when possible because being able to bang on it at strategic times seems to emphasize the solid, obvious, visceral qualities that descriptions refer to, but robust features in other sensory modalities (for example, an object with bright, vivid colors) might provide similar opportunities.

Once the client has seen the distinction between evaluative and descriptive language with respect to an emotionally neutral object, a similar process can be repeated with thoughts surrounding an emotion the client is currently experiencing.

Therapist: Okay, so from that perspective, let's take a look at the anxiety you've been experiencing and the thoughts that come along with that. Can you give me some descriptions of what your body feels like when you're anxious?

Client: My heart races. I get tense. I start to sweat.

Therapist: Good—you can feel your heart beat faster, feel your muscles tighten up, feel yourself sweating. All descriptions. What else?

Client: Well, I get nauseated sometimes. And sometimes it gets so bad that I shake.

Therapist: Okay. Now let me ask you: That muscle tension, that fast heartbeat, the sweating, the nausea—are those part of the anxiety, like properties of the anxiety, or are they something your mind adds to the anxiety?

Client: They're properties of the anxiety.

Therapist: Now let's look at some of the evaluations your mind throws out when you're anxious. I think we already have a couple— "I'm not worth getting to know," "I say dumb things." "Dumb," "unworthy"—can you grab those in the same way that you can grab this table? [*Grabs table.*]

Client: No. They always seem pretty convincing, though.

Therapist: Yeah, evaluations are pretty good at masquerading as descriptions when you're upset. But as you sit there now and look at those words—"dumb," "unworthy"—are they solid like this? [*Hits table.*]

Client: No...I guess they're really not.

Therapist: And what other kinds of thoughts—evaluations—show up when you're anxious?

Client: There's something wrong with me.

Therapist: "Wrong"—like "unacceptable"?

Client: Yeah, pretty much.

Therapist: "Unacceptable." Can you reach out and grab that?

Client: No, but I *feel* unacceptable.

Therapist: Could you reach out and hit the table with your hand a few times?

Client: [*Hits table.*]

Therapist: Can you feel "unacceptable" in the same way that you can feel this table? Can you see "unacceptable" in full color, in three dimensions, in the same way you can see this table?

Client: No. It's a tough one, though.

Therapist: Yeah. And let's just take one last look. Does "unacceptable" have the same solidity as this? [*Hits table.*]

Client: Well, uh, no.

Therapist: So what if that's all thoughts are, especially the evaluations? They're convincing, especially when you're upset, but in the end, isn't there this airy quality to them? They just don't carry the weight they pretend to....How does all this hit you?

Client: It feels like it makes sense. I'm not sure I can hold on to that perspective, though.

Therapist: Right. It takes practice, and your mind will work hard to convince you all those evaluations are true. But we'll practice over the coming sessions, as long as it's helpful.

Anxiety is a good emotion to focus this exercise on, if the client is currently experiencing it, because the physical (descriptive) and nonphysical (evaluative) aspects of anxiety are relatively easy to spot. Other emotions, of course, can be used as well. The description-evaluation exercise can walk a tightrope between defusion and restructuring. At a basic level, it appears to ask the client to place thoughts into one of two categories, and then to trust the verbal definitions of these categories as "true." In actuality, the exercise is designed to help the client notice a basic distinction between the direct, visceral experience of physically perceiving things and the indirect, ethereal nature of thoughts. And it is not a matter of descriptive language being "true" and evaluative language being "false." Rather, it is simply a matter of placing thoughts into their respective categories, and then letting the client draw on her direct, exercise-related history of noticing how solid or airy those kinds of thoughts are.

Sometimes it can be difficult to determine if a thought is an evaluation or a description. Some words are both. The word "fat," for example, refers in descriptive fashion to the presence of adipose tissue. But many people's minds might readily add evaluative baggage to the word "fat" as well. As a rule of thumb, grant the descriptive component of a word or phrase when it becomes apparent, and then ask the client what it "means" to have that word apply to him. Typically, what will emerge are a number of negatively evaluative thoughts about what it means, for example, to be "fat." These purely evaluative thoughts can then be sorted into their proper category. Even a thought like "I'm not interesting" might be said to have a descriptive component, as a client could argue that others do not show physical indications of interest toward him. In such cases, it can be helpful to grant, perhaps just for a moment, that the word or phrase is a true description of the client. Then the client can be asked what it means to "not be interesting," or what "not being interesting" says about what kind of person the client is. As in the prior example, a variety of likely negatively evaluative thoughts may then present themselves for categorization.

Finally, sometimes the kinds of problematic thoughts looked at through the description-evaluation lens are not obviously descriptive or evaluative, but rather verbal rules about how you must or must not, or should or should not, behave in particular situations. If an important verbal rule emerges during or after the exercise, it can be handled in at least two ways. Often, the client can be asked what kind of person he would be if he followed the rule, or did not follow the rule. Positive evaluative thoughts will likely arise when the client considers following the rule, and negative evaluative thoughts when he does not. Alternatively, the therapist could grant that there really do appear to be three types of thoughts: descriptions, evaluations, and rules. Rules can often pretend to be like descriptions, to describe the only way that things can or must be done. The client can then be asked what she thinks about the particular rule under consideration: Is that the only way things can be done, or might there be others? Do evaluations about following or not following the rule try to creep in and make the rule look truer? And since *those* thoughts are evaluations, how true could they possibly be?

Conclusion

Four different ways of introducing defusion in treatment for the first time have been discussed here. There are likely many, many more. While many therapists tend to have a primary strategy for their initial defusion pitch, it is wise to stay flexible. As has been stated, some defusion techniques simply do not work with some clients. Practice using some or all of these techniques. Then, if one of them falls flat, you will be prepared to move on to one of the others.

CHAPTER 6

Defusion Metaphors

Metaphors, in general, may facilitate defusion because they imply taking a more playful, less literal stance toward thoughts. They invite us to figure out how the two things being compared are similar, with a full understanding that they are in many ways not identical. An anxious client who is told that "struggling with anxiety is like struggling in quicksand" is likely to immediately see the similarity. That client is very unlikely to respond with statements like, "Yes, because the more you struggle with anxiety, the dirtier you get, and it smells like a swamp." Irrelevant features of the vehicle (what the topic of interest is compared to) are immediately discarded or not transferred to the tenor (the topic of interest). In a way, the relationship between vehicle and tenor is analogous to the relationship between thoughts and the phenomena they attempt inadequately to describe. Thoughts may capture aspects of what is really there, but are not a wholly truthful description of it. Thus, thoughts should be taken as lightly as a metaphor's vehicle.

Metaphors designed specifically to facilitate defusion often provide an overarching way of viewing the products of the mind, of building doubt about the veracity of one's thoughts. If a given metaphor produces significant defusion for a client, the metaphor can often be just briefly alluded to at later times to similar effect. Successful defusion metaphors actually change the way the client thinks. This may seem ironic, given that defusion is used to teach that thoughts do not have to be changed in order to constructively move forward. In actuality, virtually any successful defusion technique can produce new thoughts, such as "That is just a thought, and thoughts are just words." Using defusion does not deny that thought change can be helpful. It simply demonstrates how our distressing or counterproductive thoughts don't need to go away.

As with any defusion technique, some defusion metaphors will resonate with a given client and some will not. The therapist should not "push" a metaphor if it does not appear to produce any significant amount of defusion. A failed metaphor is the therapist's cue to move on to something different. In general, apt metaphors created by a client are preferable to those delivered by the therapist. The client's creation of such a metaphor means that the central message of defusion is understood and embraced; and the client will be less likely to forget something that he himself came up with.

Defusion metaphors can be brief or relatively involved comparisons. Descriptions and dialogues involving both types are included below.

The Computer Programming Metaphor

The computer programming metaphor (adapted from the "Identifying Programming" exercise in Hayes et al., 1999) compares problematic thoughts to lines programmed into a computer. One intent behind the metaphor is to highlight the historical nature of thoughts. Our past experiences, including things that people have said and done to us, "program" thoughts into our minds. When we encounter a situation that resembles one of those past experiences, our minds instantly "spit out" the relevant pieces of programming, or relevant thoughts. Whether or not the thoughts are true does not matter, and even completely arbitrary thoughts can be programmed. If they have been programmed, they will come out under the right circumstances, and thoughts that have been more frequently programmed will start to look like absolute truths. A related intent of the metaphor is to highlight the automatic and repetitive nature of thoughts, likening them to a programmed computer code that is repeatedly run when conditions are right. Thoughts seem to imply that they are a reflection of present real-world circumstances. The computer metaphor can help remind a client that many of our thoughts may simply be a reflection of our past experiences, automatically superimposing itself on our present.

The computer metaphor has some additional facets to it as well. Likening herself to a computer and her thoughts to programming creates some distance between the client and her thoughts. As will be discussed in depth in chapter 8, getting distance from thoughts is an important component of defusion. This distance can even be physicalized in session by typing one or more of the client's problematic thoughts into a computer or smartphone and having her view those thoughts from different physical perspectives (as demonstrated in the narrative below). Additionally, it can be easier for a client hearing this metaphor to see that her thoughts do not define her, just as a computer's programming does not define the computer. Regardless of what programming her mind churns out, she (like the computer) will always be there, with the same worth and potential she has always had.

The following dialogue demonstrates the use of this metaphor. Note that in many of the dialogues here and in chapters 7, 8, and 9, the "client" parts of the dialogue are relatively brief. This is a strategic move designed to give just enough information about the client to illustrate defusion techniques that are appropriately tied in to the thoughts and feelings the client is struggling with, without using too much of this book's limited space on extraneous detail.

Client: I just feel so inadequate around people…just not good enough.

Therapist: And that thought, "I'm just not good enough"—how long have you had that thought, and that feeling of inadequacy?

Client: A long time, I think. Since I was a kid.

Therapist: Can you remember one of the first times you felt that way, and believed you weren't good enough?

Client: I remember trying to help my dad restore a cabinet, when I was, I don't know, seven or eight. You know how eager you are to please grown-ups when you're a kid. But I kept messing things up, no matter how hard I tried. I remember my dad getting really frustrated, and I remember him saying, "You can't do this. Just go and play or something."

Therapist: "You can't do this." And that message—"You can't do this," "You're not good enough"—did you get that from your dad, and from others, at other times?

Client: Yes. Not all the time, but I felt like I got that vibe from a lot of people.

Therapist: Well, what if it's like this. Our minds are kind of like computers, computers that get "programmed" by our experiences. So you had that experience with your dad, and it was like he kind of typed in, regardless of whether or not he meant to, "You can't do this," "You're not good enough." And he programmed in that feeling of inadequacy. Then you had other experiences. Maybe a kid teasing you at school, or getting a bad grade on a test—and those experiences typed in, "You're not good enough." And the way this computer—the way your mind—works is that, when you're in circumstances that appear similar to those where that programming was typed in, your mind just automatically spits out those thoughts, that feeling.

Client: I mean, yeah, it does feel automatic. It makes sense that my experiences would do that to me—sort of write a program that makes those thoughts come out under the right circumstances. But how do I stop it from doing that?

Therapist: Well, that's the thing. What if once it's programmed, it's programmed? You can add new programming—maybe thoughts like, "No, I'm a good person," and maybe next time that thought will come up after "I'm not good enough" comes up. But in your experience, does that second bit of programming make "I'm not good enough" go away?

Client: No.

Therapist: Yeah, and the more you try to delete "I'm not good enough," the more new thoughts, new programming, get added. And your mind spits those out, and you don't believe the positive ones. But those negative ones…

Client: Yeah, I believe those.

Therapist: So we're stuck with the programming. But what if it's like this: I bet you've had a number of those "I'm not good enough" situations where "I'm not good enough" isn't even really true. Like, you know the kinds of things kids tease each other about, the kinds of names they call each other. Stupid things. Inaccurate things. Unfair things. Do you remember being teased about things that, in retrospect, seemed arbitrary, or unfair?

Client: Yeah, I'm sure I have. Like you said, a lot of things kids tease each other about are just stupid, unfair.

Therapist: Even that situation with your dad. You were seven, trying to refinish a cabinet. That's hard for a seven-year-old kid. In an alternate reality, maybe "I can't do this yet, but I can learn how to do it" might have been programmed in.

Client: I wish it had been.

Therapist: Yeah. But do you see what I mean? A lot of our programming can be arbitrary, or unfair, or inaccurate, or not capture the big picture. And our mind still spits that programming out in similar situations. We can't delete that programming, and we have to listen to it and feel it when it comes out, but we can notice that that programming isn't the final arbiter of what is so.

Client: It sure is convincing, though.

Therapist: Yes. Those thoughts, those feelings, have been programmed into you a lot of times. Makes it feel real, comprehensive, definitive. But what if a lot of it is arbitrary, or inaccurate, or unfair, or doesn't capture the big picture?

While the interaction depicted here could be enough to raise the client's skepticism about the veracity of his thoughts, this metaphor could be extended. The continued interaction below makes the metaphor more experiential and applies it to a few specific thoughts the client is struggling with.

The dialogue has a strong self-as-context feel to it (more will be said about the intersections between defusion and self-as-context in chapter 8), and also calls on the client to willingly accept the experiences that arise as he focuses on this one problematic thought.

Therapist: Yes. Those thoughts, those feelings, have been programmed into you a lot of times. Makes it feel real, comprehensive, definitive. But what if a lot of it is arbitrary, or inaccurate, or unfair, or doesn't capture the big picture?

Client: Maybe. But it just seems so *true*, and it feels like it's always with me—just this sense of not being good enough.

Therapist: Yeah, it feels like it's always there, like it consumes you. Can we try to look at this piece of programming from a slightly different perspective? Would it be okay if I type that thought, "I'm not good enough," on my laptop there, so we could view it a few different ways?

Client: Uh, I guess, if you think it might help.

Therapist: [*Types in "I'm not good enough."*] If you're willing, I'd like you to sit down in this chair and put your face really close to the screen, so that you can read that whole sentence but it's pretty much all that you can see.

Client: [*Puts face close to screen.*]

Therapist: What thoughts are coming up for you now?

Client: Well, it feels bad to have it front and center like that. I'm thinking, "What's the point?" and remembering some of the dumb things I've done.

Therapist: Yeah, the programming that goes along with that "I'm not good enough." Why don't you go ahead and type in "What's the point?" here as well. And maybe a specific thought about a "dumb" [*uses his fingers to mimic quotation marks in the air*] thing you did in the past, just to put those pieces of programming front and center.

Client: Okay.

Therapist: Good. If you're willing, go ahead and move in close to the screen again so that pretty much all you're seeing is those thoughts. Notice what shows up for you when they're front and center.

Client: Just…wow. More bad memories. More times when I messed things up. More times when I let people down.

Therapist: Yeah. And you can remember back to when all that programming was typed into your "computer." [*Therapist points to his own head.*] And you can imagine all those harsh, uncompromising, self-critical thoughts being programmed in back then as well. And when circumstances force that programming to pop up again and it's up close like that, it's like that's all there is. It's like that's *how* it is. Even if they weren't fair, or were just partially accurate, they feel like they completely and totally define you.

Client: I guess I don't always feel like that. But when I start thinking of those things, that's pretty much how it feels.

Therapist: Okay. Now, I'd like you to lean back in your chair and look at those thoughts, that programming, typed into your computer from a distance. Just take a look at the words and letters that make up those thoughts, and tell me what you can see. Not just the programming, but everything else you can see as you look toward that screen.

Client: Well, the computer. Your desk…the books and the bookshelves on the wall. That picture.

Therapist: As far as what's showing up for you now—what you're thinking, what you're feeling, what you're remembering— are there any differences between now and when your face was right up close to the screen?

Client: It's not as intense. I was thinking and noticing different things the second time. When I was up close, it really kind of did feel like that was all there was to me.

Therapist: And when you backed up, there was more to it than that?

Client: Yes. It's like those thoughts, those memories, are my whole world when I'm so focused on them. I forget there's more to it. Maybe I take them too seriously.

Therapist: That's what that computer—what your mind—does. It sucks you into that narrative. Makes you believe it's the Gospel, when really it's just some subjective opinions, partial perspectives, and so on that were programmed into it. If you back up from it, and notice those thoughts as thoughts, as programming, they have less of a hold over you. They don't define you.

The Passengers on the Bus Metaphor

Another classic defusion metaphor likens distressing thoughts and feelings to unwanted passengers on a bus the client is driving (Hayes et al., 1999). The metaphor incorporates several key processes central to ACT, such as values-driven action and acceptance of difficult emotions. The acceptance of difficult emotions component could be difficult to pull off successfully without an adequate understanding of how that process is addressed in ACT (discussion of which is beyond the scope of this book), so care should be taken if the metaphor is used outside an ACT context. The following dialogue demonstrates its use, and assumes the therapist is inserting thoughts and feelings that the client has previously endorsed into the narrative.

Therapist: Let's see if we can look at those thoughts and feelings you've been struggling with from a little different perspective. Imagine life is like driving a bus. At first, you enjoy it quite a bit. You drive around wherever you want to go, taking whatever turns you want to take. And then things start happening. You start making stops, at those points in your life where important things are happening, and take on passengers. Some of those passengers are those happy thoughts and feelings that you have—"I have a good wife," "I love my children," "I've got a decent job." Other passengers aren't so pretty. At one of those stops, "I'm a fraud" climbs on, and "Shame," and "Self-doubt," and "Anxiety." Those guys are ugly, scary, and intimidating. And they're on your bus.

Client: I would really, really like to kick them off.

Therapist: And my guess is you've tried that, many times. [*Compassionately.*] How has it worked?

Client: It hasn't really. Sometimes they get off, but sooner or later they're right back on.

Therapist: Yeah. And these guys, they start to dictate where you can go, what you can do—which way you can drive. For example, you might get the idea to start a new, challenging project at work, but then "Self-doubt" and "I'll fail" and "Fear" start yelling at you from the back of the bus to stop, or else. What would you typically do at that point?

Client: I probably just don't start the project.

Therapist: Yeah—those passengers are so scary and threatening that you stop the bus so that they won't come up and follow through on their threats. This may sound like an odd question, but exactly how do they threaten you? What does it seem like they'll do if they get all the way up to the front of the bus, right in your face?

Client: Well, they're just so overwhelming. They're too much to bear.

Therapist: Overwhelming—kind of like they would consume you if you let them get all the way to the front?

Client: Yes.

Therapist: And let me ask you—has there ever been a time when you let them come all the way up to the front and stay as long as they want, do whatever they want to do?

Client: No…I mean, there have been times when they weren't that strong and I was able to follow through with what I wanted to do. But when the fear and the self-doubt are strong, I do whatever I can to keep them at bay.

Therapist: So—correct me if I'm wrong here—it sounds like you've never had a chance to find out what happens when those really tough-looking passengers get all the way to the front of the bus.

Client: I guess not.

Therapist: And I'm with you. They're very scary and very intimidating. It feels like if they got there, they'd beat you up badly, overwhelm you, consume you. I know that feeling. But what if all those passengers—those thoughts and feelings—can do when they get to the front is make you look at them, Mmke you hear the thoughts and the threats and feel the feelings?

Client: But is that what it's like?

Therapist: In my experience, yeah. With tough thoughts and feelings, it's tough—it's painful. But wouldn't it be worth it to risk experiencing that if it meant that you could take back control of the wheel, and do the things you really want to be doing in your life?

This metaphor can be augmented by being physically acted out. Once the client's key distressing thoughts and feelings are identified, the client is asked to engage in a task (inside or outside the therapist's office, as possible) she would like to engage in. After asking permission from the client to do so, the therapist then acts as the passengers, reciting the respective thoughts and emotions and elaborating objections intended to stop the client from engaging in her chosen task. To make the task more meaningful, the client can designate an object or destination as symbolic of a specific, important, and meaningful course of action she would like to take in life. Then the task can involve interacting with that object or walking toward that destination despite the client's "passengers" voicing their objections. Physicalizing this metaphor might seem silly, but such metaphors can often be better understood experientially. Talking about driving in a desired direction may not be as productive as actually "driving" in that direction. And the delivery of the physicalized metaphor does not have to come off as odd as one might think. A colleague of mine (Joseph Ciarrochi) actually implemented a group version of this physicalized metaphor in a training for the New South Wales police force in which an officer volunteered to "drive his own bus" while the other officers enthusiastically shouted out his doubts and fears.

Carry Your Keys

In this metaphor, defusion, acceptance, values, and self-as-context are combined to illustrate how it can often be necessary to experience distressing thoughts and feelings while acting in accordance with your values. The metaphor is simple. Once you have identified core thoughts and feelings that make it difficult for the client to engage in one or more valued actions, ask the client to produce her keychain. The following dialogue demonstrates what might happen next.

Therapist: [*Holding the keychain.*] What's useful about this?

Client: About my keychain? Uh….Well, I couldn't drive my car without it.

Therapist: What else?

Client: I couldn't go home—unlock my apartment. My office key is on there, too, so I couldn't go to work—which wouldn't be bad. [*Laughs.*]

Therapist: Good. I'm with you on that one! I'm not happy about going to work some days either. Why do you go to work, then?

Client: Well, money, of course.

Therapist: For what?

Client: To live—pay for my rent, for my kids' clothes and stuff.

Therapist: Including things like presents, nice things for your family.

Client: Yes.

Therapist: And why do you do that?

Client: Well, I love them.

Therapist: Yeah, we've talked a bit about that. About how important it is to you to provide for them, take care of them, let them have the kind of childhood and parents that you didn't get to have. Let me ask you this: Those days that you go to work, and you really don't want to, what do you feel like? What kinds of things do you think?

Client: I just feel…burdened, harried. I wish I could call in sick. I think, "Here we go again—another long week doing stuff that I hate."

Therapist: And yet you still go. Well, let's look at this a bit differently. Which one is your office key? This one? [*Holds key.*] This represents your values with respect to Ava and Emma. [*Best to use her children's actual names to emphasize the personal elements of the value.*] This key opens that door. I know you don't normally equate your office with your love for your children, but it sounds like that's why you go to work every day. Am I right?

Client: Yes. I almost don't want to connect my kids to work, but that's mainly why I do it.

Therapist: Yeah. And these other keys are the feelings and thoughts that show up when you think about going to work. This one's "Burdened." This one here is "Harried." This one is "I want to call in sick." This one is "Another day doing what I hate." Would you be willing to take your keys back at this point and just hold on to them and look at them?

Client: At this point, I'm not sure. I've never thought of my keys like that before.

Therapist: I hear you. There's stuff here that you don't want to have. And yet it sounds like, almost every weekday, you take these feelings and thoughts [*points to a few individual keys*] to work with you, because of this [*displays office key*]: because of your love for your kids, because of what you want to provide for them. [*Keeps holding on to office key and offers key ring again to client.*] Would you be willing to take it by this key, and then we can take a look at the other keys?

Client: Okay. [*Takes key ring by office key.*]

Therapist: And let's look at those other keys again. Show me "Burdened"…"Harried"…"Another long day at a job I hate"…"I wish I could call in sick." If it means that you get to provide some of those things, those experiences, that you really want for Ava and Emma, would you be willing to carry those keys—those thoughts and feelings—with you? Because you could leave that whole key ring behind if you wanted to.

Client: [*Pauses.*] Okay, I see what you mean. I could stop going to work because I hate it, but then that would mean I couldn't provide a lot of things I want to provide for Ava and Emma.

Therapist: Right. And if you're willing to carry all the keys on that ring, it means that you get that key that opens up those opportunities.

Client: Hmm. I go to work most of the time anyway, but I've never thought about it like this before. Yes, of course I'm willing to carry it.

Therapist: Good. Now let's extend this a bit. I know you've mentioned that it's also very important to you that you're kind and loving, toward your children. That you really connect with them, rather than just detaching. What kinds of thoughts and feelings get in the way of you doing those things consistently?

Client: Well, feeling tired—burned out from work. Sometimes I just want to tune out at home and I get frustrated or annoyed with their questions, with things that they're doing. And I think, "I just need a break."

Therapist: Okay, so we've got that values key again—that one that corresponds to loving, supporting, and connecting with your children. Can you show that one to me? Cool. And let's label the other keys. That next one…that's "Feeling burned out." The next one—"Feeling tired." And that one is "Frustration." And that one—"I just need a break." Would you be willing to carry those with you if it meant that you could really connect with Ava and Emma, really be there for them?

Client: I don't know if I could do it all the time, but I could do it more.

Therapist: Good, yes. We're not talking all the time here. Just as a moment-to-moment choice, could you carry those thoughts and feelings—those keys—with you and still open the door to that connection, rather than those other keys preventing that from happening?

This metaphor is typically applied immediately to a constellation of thoughts and feelings that often work to "prevent" valued action (as demonstrated in the dialogue when the metaphor is extended to the client's experience of trying to connect with her children after a busy work day). The first part of the dialogue illustrates how fortuitous circumstances (in this case, the client already showing a capacity to act consistently with a child-related value at one level by going to work regularly, even with difficult thoughts and feelings) can be capitalized on and extended. Clients tend to "get" the metaphor at a visceral level. Keys open doors and allow you to go places. If you don't take them with you, the opportunity to get there is closed. Other thoughts and feelings will come along for the ride, but they can be willingly carried *as* thoughts and feelings if it means the valued journey can continue.

The Master Storyteller

This metaphor (adapted from Harris, 2009) likens the mind to a masterful and creative storyteller. As with most great storytellers, the mind begins its story as nonfiction, but quickly embellishes and creates a compelling story that never really happened—at least not precisely the way it was told. The brief dialogue below represents one possible application.

Therapist: The mind works kind of like a master author or storyteller might. It starts off telling a story that looks like nonfiction. It starts by reporting the facts, setting the scene. And then, even though those facts could form the basis for any number of different stories, it starts to weave them together into one specific narrative. And seamlessly, embellishments and interpretations start getting thrown in alongside the facts. Eventually, the story becomes so compelling that you can't imagine it being a different story. It becomes so engrossing that it seems absolutely true. We'll use an example. Who is one of your favorite fiction authors?

Client: Uh…well, I really like Hemingway. *The Sun Also Rises*, *The Old Man and the Sea*.

Therapist: Okay. And what do you like best about Hemingway?

Client: Well, to borrow your phrase, he's really good at setting a scene. Like a reporter—he has a really sparse writing style, but you know where they are, what the characters are like.

Therapist: And the human element of his books—do you feel for the characters? Do they feel like real-life situations?

Client: Some more than others. I really got drawn in by the guy in *The Old Man and the Sea*.

Therapist: I remember that book—not being able to put it down, worrying about him, really hoping he'd make it first of all, and then hoping he'd bring that big fish in.

Client: Yeah—me, too. It was great.

Therapist: And it was like it was real, right? I mean, you step away from it and at some point you remember it's fiction. But it's so human, so realistically dramatic—you're so aware that something exactly like this really could happen.

Client: Yeah, I almost do forget sometimes that his books are fiction.

Therapist: And what if our minds work like that? We survey the situation we're in, set the scene. And then our minds start weaving that narrative, filling in the gaps, sometimes creating motivations for other characters in our lives. Piling interpretations and judgments of the main character [*nods to client*] and the other characters on top of that. Creating a story so compelling that it's not just *a* story, it's *the* story—*the* account of what actually happened, with no errors or omissions.

Client: I guess I can see that. I know sometimes I look back on things I've told myself—or, I guess, that my mind has told me—that seem kind of dramatic. But it doesn't feel that way in the moment, like when I'm really focused on something that really bothers me.

Therapist: And that's the trick of a good novelist, right? Knowing how to hook you so well that you don't even question the truth of what's written on that page. And your mind knows you very, very well. It knows what hooks you, the story lines and the judgments that grab hold of you, better than anyone. It's like the ultimate, personalized novelist. It knows how to write a book that is very hard for you to put down.

Client: Very hard. In fact, in the moment, how do I put it down?

Therapist: I think you already took the first step: acknowledging that not everything your mind says is true. From there, we'll do a number of things in therapy [*implicitly referring to other defusion techniques*] from here on out to help you put that book down when you need to.

You can imagine using this metaphor with a variety of authors and genres, even those with books based in fantastical settings. While many of us read far-fetched books to temporarily escape from our day-to-day lives, most of us are also very engaged by the human element of a story. We like characters we care about, and are moved by events that evoke strong emotions and honest reactions in those characters, by their tragedies and triumphs. This is a big part of what makes a story compelling and believable, and it is what makes our own stories compelling and believable. Pointing out this dynamic in a work of fiction can help a client question whether his mind might be going beyond "setting the scene" and providing some of the same compelling embellishments a master storyteller might provide.

Thoughts as Hands

The "Thoughts as Hands" metaphor (adapted from Harris, 2009) uses a simple physical metaphor to illustrate how buying into our problematic thoughts obscures our view of the world around us, convincing us that those thoughts define reality. The client is asked to liken her thoughts to her hands, and to contrast her experience of the world when her hands are right in front of her face versus farther away. The following dialogue demonstrates an individualized adaptation of the metaphor.

> Client: I just worry about everything. I worry about my kids getting hurt, worry about my job, about keeping my head above water, about whether or not I'll get any sleep at night.

> Therapist: It's like the worry is almost always there. Can I ask what kinds of thoughts show up when you're worried? Like when you're worried about your kids getting hurt, for example.

> Client: Well, I think, what if their bus crashed on the way to school or the way back? What if a bully is beating one of them up right now? What if they start using drugs, or drinking? What if they get hurt playing?

Therapist: Okay. Am I right in guessing that at those times, those thoughts are front and center? That it's hard to think about anything else?

Client: Yes. That happens regardless of what I'm worrying about at a given moment. It's hard to think about anything else.

Therapist: Well, let's try something. Go ahead and hold your hand out in front of you. Just to get a glimpse into what this process looks like, let's label each of your fingers, one by one, with those thoughts. So, your thumb, that's "What if the bus crashed?" Your pointer finger—"What if a bully is beating them up?" Next finger—"What if they start using drugs?" Next one—"What if they get hurt playing?" And I imagine there are a number of other worrisome thoughts that could fill up both of your hands, right?

Client: Definitely.

Therapist: Now, I'd like you to put your hands together, palms up, side by side, fingers close together. And orient again toward those thoughts you labeled your fingers with....Now put your hands right in front of your eyes, so they're almost touching your face. What do you see?

Client: Just part of my fingers and my hands. I can see off to the sides a little bit, but not much.

Therapist: And those thoughts that you labeled your fingers with...is this what it's like when you're focused on thoughts like that? Like those thoughts are pretty much your world, like you can't see or think about anything else?

Client: Yes—it is pretty much like this.

Therapist: And your worried thoughts about other things—is it the same process there? They come up, completely take over the view, like there's almost nothing else there?

Client: Yes, usually I can hardly think about anything else.

Therapist: My guess is they don't even look like thoughts at those points, just as your fingers don't exactly look like fingers at that distance. Do they seem like a commentary on reality, like that's just what's really there?

Client: Yeah, they do. I've been able to notice some of my thoughts as thoughts since I started seeing you, but the worried ones— it's like that's just how it is.

Therapist: Okay. And I'd like you to notice how hampered you are right now, how disabled you are with your hands right in front of your eyes. How good of a job do you think you could do walking around the room, or driving home, or getting things done at home, with your hands like that?

Client: Not a good job at all. I doubt if I could even get to the door without tripping on something.

Therapist: Right. And how effective are you when you're holding those worrisome thoughts close, taking them for granted?

Client: Well, I can usually get to a door without tripping, but sometimes I get so distracted that I can't do much of anything.

Therapist: Exactly. When you don't even notice them as thoughts, you hold them close. Sometimes you can't even see enough of the world around you to function. Let's try something else. Move your hands away from your face, maybe about two feet in front of you, and spread your fingers open. Good. Now let's physically label some of those fingers again, one by one. What were the thoughts about your kids?

Client: What if they're using drugs? What if the bus crashed? What if they get hurt playing? What if they're being bullied?

Therapist: Good. And as you look at your hands now, what do you see?

Client: Well, I still see my hands and my fingers.

Therapist: Right. Those thoughts are still there, aren't they? And what's different this time—what else can you see?

Client: I can see pretty much everything in the room. My hands and fingers block a little bit from here, but not much.

Therapist: Good. You've tagged those thoughts as thoughts, gotten some distance. They're still there, but you can see more of the world around you. More possibilities.

Client: But I still worry. It still bothers me to worry that they could be hurt right now.

Therapist: Right—just like those fingers, your hands, are still there. It doesn't get rid of the worry, the thoughts. But is noticing those thoughts—those fingers—a bit different from when they were right up against your eyes?

Client: A bit.

Therapist: I want to ask something else, too. When those worrisome thoughts come up, it looks to me like they're very compelling, they just seem like facts. Is that right?

Client: Yes—that's why I worry so much when they come up.

Therapist: So one advantage of noticing them as thoughts, out there, is that it gives you the opportunity to contrast them with your direct experience. For example, how many times has your kids' bus crashed?

Client: Never, but that doesn't mean it won't crash.

Therapist: You're right. It could. But notice how quickly and closely that thought, "What if their bus has crashed?" has grabbed you in the past. It presents itself as a simple reflection of reality, as something that's imminent, likely to happen. And your experience says it's never happened to your kids yet, but it could happen. If it's up here [*holds his hands in front of his own face*], it's the whole world. Nothing else is out there. If it's out here [*holds his hands a few feet away, fingers spread open*], it's just a thought. And once they're out here, your direct experience about what *has* happened gets to have some input.

Client: I get what you're saying. I just worry I won't be able to remember this when I need to.

Therapist: It will take practice, but I'll help you point out thoughts like these regularly as we go along.

This metaphor can be used in a more general form, without labeling individual fingers with problematic thoughts, but this dialogue demonstrates how personalizing it can provide the client with a more in-depth experience. Having the client physically label several fingers with distressing thoughts can help her get some distance from thoughts that normally automatically color her perception of her experience. As the exercise becomes more specific, it also gives her more opportunity to disagree or qualify her reactions—which in turn provides the therapist more opportunity to constructively address those reactions.

Conclusion

A good metaphor can quickly help us view our experiences from a markedly different perspective. Defusion metaphors can serve as a way of introducing defusion, building on earlier defusion work, or (when a client embraces a particular metaphor) providing a way to talk about unhooking from thoughts on an ongoing basis. The five metaphors discussed in this chapter can serve any of these purposes. Many other defusion metaphors have been developed by therapists over the years (see, for example, Stoddard & Afari, 2014). And as with other types of defusion techniques, you should always be ready to capitalize on client-generated metaphors.

CHAPTER 7

Changing Language Parameters

The sentences we think and speak make sense only if certain rules are followed. Grammar must be used correctly, or at least reasonably correctly. Words, and the letters that make them up, must be ordered in a particular fashion. The definitions of the words used must be known to the person thinking or hearing them. Marked changes to any or all of these language parameters can alter the meaning of a sentence, make you more skeptical of the veracity of the sentence (or of words in general), or even make it completely nonsensical (see, for example, Blackledge, 2007).

But these grammatical, syntactical, and semantic parameters are not the only things that affect the meaning of words. The tone and manner in which words are spoken must also reasonably match the "intended" emotive qualities attached to those words. A person earnestly expressing his sadness might likely speak in a heavy tone, and a bit more slowly than usual. Speaking the same words in a happy, excited, up-tempo fashion would cast the words differently. Additionally, sentences only make sense if spoken at a particular rate. If they are spoken too fast or too slowly, the sounds that make up each individual word start to become the prime focus of attention, and the meaning recedes into the background. Finally, thoughts sung in a particular musical style, or used as the lyrics to the melody of a particular song, can pick up some of the characteristics of that music and perhaps lose some of their original characteristics. For example, singing a sad thought in an over-the-top operatic voice might make you view the thought as more melodramatic, or might simply introduce a level of oddity that breaks up or diminishes some of the distressing or debilitating functions of the thought. Speaking a troublesome thought in the voice of a famous cartoon, movie, or television character can also markedly change how that thought is viewed. Try, for example, speaking one of your own thoughts, distressing or not, in the voice of Mickey Mouse, or in Christian Bale's Batman voice. Chances are it will significantly change the way you perceive that thought. Characters or singing styles that convey a mood quite incongruous with the initial mood a thought conveys, or that impart a sense of absurdity or humor, are typically best for this purpose.

The most central language parameter that gives words meaning involves focusing on the content those words convey, as opposed to focusing on the process of forming and speaking those words. When we have a running verbal narrative about the events in our lives, we are typically not even aware that we are "having thoughts" about those events. We have the impression that we are simply describing what those events are and how they are impacting us. We are focused completely on the content of those thoughts, usually with little or no awareness of the process of physically forming and speaking those words or of mentally observing movement from one thought to the next. Focusing on the process of thinking or speaking distracts us from fully absorbing the content of those thoughts, which in turn changes or disrupts the effect those words have on us. It can also lead us to be more suspicious of our thoughts. Once you start to notice the process of producing the letters and words that make up your thoughts, you may start to realize that thoughts aren't simply perfect reflections created by the world around and inside you. Rather, you start to see words as man-made, as fallible as the people who create them. While arguably all effective techniques of defusion (and, for that matter, of self-as-context) ultimately push our attention away from the content of our thoughts and toward the process of producing them, some defusion techniques are explicitly intended to do so. The "mind" and "thought" language discussed in chapter 5 is a good example. Several other examples of shifting attention from content to the process of producing words will be discussed later in this chapter.

As you may have already guessed, changing many of the language parameters discussed above requires a good amount of empathy and prudent delivery on the part of the therapist. Otherwise, an earnestly disclosing client may feel put off or invalidated. And as a rule of thumb, the therapist should have already used some defusion techniques and rationales with a client before using some of the more dramatic or invasive techniques described in this chapter. Many detailed ways of defusing by changing language parameters are illustrated in the dialogues below. Some of these techniques are brief and easily inserted into a conversation; their use will simply be described rather than conveyed as a dialogue.

Brief Methods of Changing Language Conventions

There are several language conventions that can be quickly used to draw a client's attention to the fact that he is thinking, rather than simply reacting to reality. (All of the following ones are adapted from Hayes et al., 1999.) Many of them can be used repeatedly within and across sessions, just as the "mind" and "thought" language discussed in chapter 5. A client might be asked to "hold a thought lightly," rather than holding on to it tightly and fully believing in it. This phrase can be used in a "one shot" fashion by targeting a single thought, as in, "Okay, let's hold that thought lightly." Or the physical nature of the metaphor can be emphasized with a series of thoughts, as in, "Let's watch each thought that comes up and just sort of touch it lightly." Alternatively, you can talk in terms of "buying a thought" or "not buying a thought." "I'm not buying it" is a long-standing American English idiom for "I don't believe it," making the notion of buying or not buying thoughts readily accessible to any client who has heard the idiom. A third change of phrase, the *and-but* convention, involves asking the client to substitute the word "and" for the word "but" when a client utters a sentence that involves a state of affairs that seems to preclude a desired action, as demonstrated below.

Client: I've just burned too many bridges. I haven't talked to my kids for over six years. I don't think they even want to talk to me, after all the problems I've caused. I really want to see them, but I feel so ashamed.

Therapist: Yeah, I can see how hopeless it must feel to really want to connect with them, and to feel like there's no chance. I want to look at that last thought, though: "I really want to see them, but I feel so ashamed." The word "but" is a tricky one in thoughts like this. You know, if we go back several hundred years, the word "but" was actually two words: "be out." As if you want to do something, but another thing literally has to "be out" of the way for you to be able to do it. Like here: you want to see your kids, but your mind is saying that shame needs to "be out" of the way, gone, first. I know the shame is big—you feel a lot of it, and it's very hard to have. And…is it literally physically preventing you from seeing your kids?

Client: I guess not. I just don't know if I can bear it.

Therapist: And that's something we'll keep working on, since it clearly matters to you that you see your kids. And for right now, I'd like to try something. As we talk for the rest of the session [*or for the next several minutes*], every time the word "but" comes up, for both of us, let's replace "but" with the word "and," and repeat the sentence. Could you try that with, "I really want to see my kids, but I feel so ashamed"?

Client: I really want to see my kids, *and* I feel so ashamed.

Therapist: Does that thought hit you any differently?

Client: A little. It's like, maybe both things can be there at the same time.

Therapist: Yeah. Maybe you could feel ashamed *and* see your kids.

The *and-but* technique may not have a dramatic effect, but it can form an opening that helps the client more seriously consider whether both conditions can coexist. When applied repeatedly over a portion of a session (or perhaps even an entire session), that opening can widen. The awkwardness of repeatedly pausing a discussion to note that a "but" was used and to rephrase the sentence can provide an added benefit, as it increases the focus on the process of speaking. The client becomes more aware that the words he uses, or "buys into," shape the way he perceives his situation.

Word Translation

An online translator such as Google Translate (or your knowledge of a foreign language) can be used to highlight the odd and arbitrary nature of a particularly powerful word and give the client a different experience with it. The process simply involves translating a key word or two from a client's distressing or counterproductive thought into a language the client is not familiar with, and then asking the client to repeat the sentence with the foreign word(s) inserted. For example, a client caught up in the thought, "I'm hopeless" might be asked to say, "I'm sin esperanza," using the Spanish words for "hopeless." The experiment can be introduced and processed as follows:

Client: I'm hopeless.

Therapist: [*Empathetically.*] Yeah…hopeless. That's a powerful word, isn't it? I mean, it's one of those words that can just completely take over. Completely make it look like there is absolutely, categorically is no hope. Does it feel like that when you say, "I'm hopeless"?

Client: Yes, yes it does.

Therapist: Let's try something here. That word "hopeless" claims that every part of you is hopeless. We could argue with it, try to build a case against it, but I know you've already done a lot of that—and the word, the thought, is still there. Let's look at that word from a little different angle, just to see if maybe there's something a little fishy about it. Do you know any Spanish?

Client: Spanish? Uh, no, not really. Just maybe a few words— *si, adios amigo*—that kind of thing.

Therapist: Okay. Let's find the Spanish word for hopeless on the computer. [*Types in word to online translator.*] *Sin esperanza.* Would you say that for me? "I'm sin esperanza."

Client: Okay—I'm sin esperanza. [*Chuckles.*] It kind of sounds like I'm giving myself a girl's name.

Therapist: Yeah. [*Laughs with client.*] "I'm sin esperanza." "Sin esperanza" claims to define your entire life. Do you believe her?

Client: [*Laughs.*] No. No, not at all.

Therapist: And that word in English makes the same claim. Different letters, different sounds, but still "sin esperanza." Sound a little bit fishy?

Client: Kind of. I really have felt completely hopeless when I've thought about that in the past. But it doesn't feel so complete right now. It's like, maybe I'm not completely hopeless.

Therapist: "I'm not completely sin esperanza"?

Client: [*Chuckles.*] Yeah…I'm not completely sin esperanza.

Therapist: [*In an attempt to remind the client that it is not necessary to change or get rid of the initial thought.*] And, you know what, my guess is "I'm hopeless" or "I'm completely hopeless" [*using fingers to make quotation marks around "completely" in the air*] is going to come back sooner or later. I want you to remember the fishiness of that "hopeless" word. "Sin esperanza." It makes a big, sweeping, definitive claim. And when you peel back those letters and look behind them… what does it look like?

Client: It just seems…suspect.

Therapist: Good.

It is advisable to look for a foreign language that yields a word the client will view as odd, almost unpronounceable, or that will otherwise create an impression (as it did in the dialogue above) far removed from the client's native-language version of the word. The ability of "sin esperanza" to invoke the image of a girl, for a non-Spanish speaker, rather than a sense of hopelessness, suggests the arbitrary nature of words. As another example, the Polish word for "hopeless" is "beznadziejny"—a word difficult to pronounce by someone with no background in Slavic languages. The physical features of that latter word, rather than its meaning, then become most prominent. It should be noted that multiple repetitions of the translated word or phrase can make the client explicitly aware of the functional equivalence of it and the native-language word. After all, this is how foreign languages are learned. Highlighting the sense of fishiness, suspiciousness, or excessive authoritativeness of the word's claims, as was done in the dialogue, can help counteract this potential outcome.

Word Repetition

The word-repetition exercise (often referred to as the "milk" exercise; Hayes et al., 1999), which I hope you engaged in while reading chapter 1, involves excessive repetition of a word. The process is intended to experientially highlight the arbitrary nature of words and reduce their literal functions. While the client is discussing distressing issues, the therapist extracts a word that more or less captures the essence of the distress and suggests replacing it with a neutral word, such as "milk." After providing a brief rationale for the exercise and having the client repeat the word "milk" quickly for about thirty seconds, the therapist asks the client to notice what thoughts, feelings, and other experiences show up when the client speaks the word that is particularly painful for her. That personalized word is then repeated just as the word "milk" was, and the client's reactions are processed. The "milk" portion of the exercise can optionally be skipped. Retaining it may make the exercise less intrusive, however, since it can help the client become familiar with the experience through the use of a word that has no strong emotional component. The exercise is exemplified below, and can be conducted in a way similar to the translation exercise above.

Client: And like I've been saying, I just feel like a complete failure in relationships. Sometimes I don't even see the point in trying to meet someone again.

Therapist: That's a painful thought to have. "Failure." Can I ask what it feels like when that word shows up?

Client: Ashamed…sad…embarrassed.

Therapist: It's a powerful word—it makes sense that all those feelings would show up. And I know that your past experiences and that "failure" thought are holding you back from trying again. I'd like to take a closer look at that word, to see if we can find a different way to hold it. Would you be willing to do that on the chance that it might help you get out in the dating pool again?

Client: I'll try anything at this point.

Therapist: Good. We've talked a bit before about how words are tricky—about how binding they can be. I want to do an exercise where we shake that up a little bit—experience that word "failure" differently. To make it a little safer, we'll do the exercise first with a neutral word—one that doesn't come with all those tough feelings—and then try it again with "failure."

Client: Okay.

Therapist: Okay. So the neutral word is "milk." Could you say that out loud and tell me what images or thoughts show up?

Client: Milk. I mean, I'm thinking about milk.

Therapist: Can you picture a glass of milk? Feel the coldness of it? Almost taste it?

Client: Yes. I'm thinking of cows now, too.

Therapist: Fine. Notice how all of that is showing up psychologically… and there isn't even any milk in the room. It's like a word has the power to bring things into the room—things that aren't even really there.

Client: Okay.

Therapist: Now this part is a bit silly, so I'll do it with you. We're going to say the word "milk" out loud fast for about thirty seconds, and see what happens. Are you okay with that?

Client: Umm…yeah, I guess so.

Therapist: Good. Ready?

[Client and therapist say "milk" repeatedly for thirty seconds; therapist periodically prompts client to say the word louder and faster if necessary.]

Therapist: Okay—stop. By the end of the exercise, what was showing up for you when you said milk?

Client: Nothing. It was just weird.

Therapist: So, no glass of milk, no cows, no coldness?

Client: No—all gone.

Therapist: Did you find yourself noticing what the word sounded like— sort of like MALK—or what it felt like to make the word's sounds?

Client: Yeah—I did. That's really all that was there.

Therapist: That's really all that words are. Just sounds strung together, movements in your mouth and throat. Or if it's written down, it's just scratches on paper. Many hundreds of years ago some guy made up that word, "milk," and everybody decided what the word would refer to. When you use the word normally, it gains the power to bring things into the room that aren't even there. But when you experience that word differently, like we just did, what happens?

Client: Well, it—yeah, it just lost all that. It's like the word was complete nonsense.

Therapist: And do you see what I mean? *All* words are like that. Just sounds. Just scratches on paper. And then we take them seriously. And then they get powerful and convince us that they are absolutely true.

Client: Yeah, I see what you mean.

Therapist: And that word, "failure." Would you be willing to say that word once again and tell me what shows up for you?

Client: Failure. The same as always. I feel ashamed, embarrassed, sad, like there's something wrong with me. Hopeless.

Therapist: Yeah. Pretty powerful, isn't it?

Client: Yes.

Therapist: And to see what happens with that word, would you be willing to say it out loud fast for about thirty seconds with me?

Client: [*Sighs.*] Yes, I can do that.

[Therapist and client repeat "failure" out loud fast for thirty seconds, with therapist prompting client to say it more quickly and louder to highlight the word's auditory and somatic properties.]

Therapist: Okay—stop. What was showing up for you toward the end of the exercise?

Client: We got to the point where we couldn't even say the word— my lips got all tied up.

Therapist: What else?

Client: Like with "milk"—the only things there were these weird sounds, my lips moving, my throat…

Therapist: Yeah. And the sadness, embarrassment, shame, hopelessness?

Client: It's still there when I think about the word. It's just kind of… different. Like it's not quite as big right now as it usually feels.

Therapist: Yeah. And I'm wondering about some of the things that word typically brings into the room, like "There's something wrong with me" because of past failures, or that finding anyone in the future is "hopeless." Because the feelings are really there, right? "Failure" doesn't bring those into the room—or maybe it brings more of those feelings. But when it has that power—do you think maybe it brings that sense of "Something is really wrong with me," "My relationship future is hopeless," into the room?

Client: But I really do feel like there is something wrong with me.

Therapist: Yeah. And those are words too, right? I wonder what would happen if we did that exercise with every one of those words, too?

Client: [*Laughs.*] That would be weird.

Therapist: Yes. And would you guess that the same thing would happen?

Client: Yeah, I think it would.

Therapist: Well, see if this rings true for you: Given the experience you just had with "milk" and "failure," is it possible that all the claims words make about what's real and what's here are overblown? That when we take some of those words seriously, they can convince us of things that may not be so?

Client: Yeah, I can see that. Like when I feel hopeless about the future, I really feel hopeless, but maybe it's not. Maybe it's just a thought. How could I really know?

Therapist: Right. Maybe words like that are taking you for a ride—but when you look at them from a different angle, they look kind of sketchy.

If the exercise is processed this way, part of the trick involves distinguishing between client experiences that are already "in the room" and additional experiences that the word "brings into the room" when it is taken literally. This particular client is likely to experience feelings like sadness, embarrassment, and pessimism as a direct result of a history of failed relationships. If the therapist claimed that the word "failure" was the *only* source of all those aspects of his experience, the client might balk and move to defend various aspects of his "failure" narrative. In contrast, framing the overreaching implications of the word "failure"—that there is something seriously wrong with him, and that his dating future is hopeless—as being "pulled into the room" by the word allows the client to more quickly understand how personally distressing words "create" psychological experiences just as a simple word like "milk" does. While other verbally mediated aspects of this client's shame and embarrassment (for example) would likely need to be confronted later in therapy, restricting the processing to certain aspects of this mediation can quickly make the client more suspicious of his thoughts.

Having Thoughts

Repeated use of the "having a thought" technique (Hayes et al., 1999) can have an even more dramatic effect in centering the client's attention on the fact that she is producing thoughts, not just verbally reflecting realities. This simple intervention involves inserting the phrase "I'm having the thought that…" in front of potentially every sentence the client speaks for a certain period of time. It can be particularly effective in slowing a client down when she is enmeshed with the content of a running narrative about the difficulties in her life. I have used this technique with as few as one or two sentences, and (very rarely) for as long as fifteen or twenty minutes. As with some other defusion techniques, lengthy use of this practice can seem awkward. But that awkwardness is part of the reason why it can be effective in helping the client to focus more on the process of creating thoughts, and to be less bound by the content of those thoughts.

> *Client:* And it's been like this for almost twenty years. I just can't pull myself up out of it. I've tried everything I can think of, but I can't make it work. I'm hopeless, and I'll always be hopeless. It's just senseless. There's no point in trying to improve myself, because I just can't do it.

> *Therapist:* I hear you. It's been like this for a long, long time. I'm wondering maybe if we can slow this down a bit. You seem to be trapped by all those thoughts. Would you be willing to look at them from a little different perspective, so that maybe we can make some room?

Client: I guess so. What perspective?

Therapist: Well, there can be a danger in taking every one of our thoughts at face value. If you're willing, I'd like you to continue telling me about the situation you're in. But this time, I'd like you to say, "I'm having the thought that…" before each sentence you speak.

Client: I don't see how that's going to get me out of this. I've been thinking this way for a long time.

Therapist: I hear you. And it probably won't change those thoughts. But it might change how you look at them. Are you willing to give it a try?

Client: Okay.

Therapist: Good. So, you were talking about how things feel hopeless, about how you can't make things in your life work.

Client: I can't. I mean, I was telling you earlier about how much I messed up that talk with my wife. I…

Therapist: Okay—let me interrupt you. Can you say, "I'm having the thought that I really messed up that talk with my wife"?

Client: I'm having the thought that I really messed up that talk with my wife.

Therapist: And if you could preface the next thought with "I'm having the thought that…"

Client: But I really did…I mean, I'm having the thought that I really did mess things up with my wife. I shouldn't have been so hard…

Therapist: And that thought, too.

Client: I'm having the thought that I shouldn't have been so hard on her.

Therapist: And the next one?

Client: I'm having the thought that I always do this....I'm having the thought that I don't understand why she's still with me.

Therapist: Good.

Client: I'm having the thought that I'm not good enough for her....I'm having the thought that I'm not good enough for anything.

Therapist: Okay.

At a point like this, a therapist could go in one of several directions, depending on which therapeutic model is being used and the nature of the client's thoughts and emotions. For example, an ACT therapist might continue using the "having a thought" convention if it still looked like the client was largely fused with the content of his thoughts. If values-related thoughts emerged (for instance, "I want to do more for my wife") or were prompted by the therapist, that path could be explored. If not, the therapist could use the opportunity to help the client more fully experience his emotions, using defusion and other core ACT processes to facilitate the process. You might consider practicing this technique with a series of your own personally distressing thoughts to gain insight into what the process feels like, and the degree of defusion it can result in. Then you may be more prepared to respond effectively to client reactions.

Slow Speech and Silly Voices

As mentioned at the beginning of the chapter, dramatically altering one's rate of speech (Hayes et al., 1999) or speaking or singing a thought (Hayes & Strosahl, 2004) in a voice or style markedly inconsistent with the content of a troublesome thought can result in defusion. Practically speaking, it is simpler to get a client to speak at a reliably slow versus sufficiently fast rate. Rationales similar to those listed in the dialogues above can be used to introduce the endeavor. The rate of speech should be very slow—I timed myself at about two seconds per syllable, though I typically count quickly to five in my head to pace how long to draw out a syllable when using this technique. Speaking more quickly than that tends to retain too much of the words' meanings.

Obviously, a great variety of "silly" voices (or, more precisely, voices discordant with the content of the words being spoken), singing styles, or songs can be used to facilitate defusion. Guidelines for what kinds of voices, singing styles, or songs to use were given early in this chapter. A number of voice-changing apps are available for Android, iPhone, and Windows smartphones. These apps temporarily record whatever you say and then play it back in an altered voice. Applications like "Voice Changer," "Ultra Voice Changer," and "Simple Voice Changer" on Android are good examples, and are all currently available for free. Some of the higher-rated voice-changing apps for iPhones include "Voicemod," "Voice Lab," and "Voices 2." Well-regarded Windows Phone voice apps include "Voice Changer" and "Fun Voice." Software apps such as "MorphVOX" for PC and "MorphVOX Mac Voice Changer" for Apple computers are available as well, but are markedly more expensive than their mobile app counterparts. Applications like these have many preset options (for example, "chipmunk," "robot," and "helium" voices) that may dramatically change the tone and pitch of a recorded voice. Searching for any of these titles in your app store will reveal dozens of similar apps, though it should be noted that many of these do not change voices markedly enough to facilitate defusion. It is advisable to test any app you recommend for a client first, and even help the client find the voice settings within the chosen app that seem to produce higher degrees of defusion for him.

Rearranging Thoughts

So far in this chapter, we have focused largely on techniques that alter the way thoughts are spoken and heard. Violating language parameters that govern the meaningful presentation of written words can also result in defusion. You can ask your client to "write" a troublesome thought on a table using letter tiles, such as those used in Scrabble (sets of replacement Scrabble tiles can be purchased online to reduce cost). Normally, we don't "construct" thoughts in our minds by building them letter by letter. Thoughts typically emerge as complete entities, almost spontaneously. Thus, the extended act of deliberately searching for each tile and spelling out the thought, letter by letter, can by itself significantly change how we relate to our thoughts. Once the sentence is spelled correctly, ask the client to rearrange the letters several times to form both new words and meaningless strings of letters. Finally, ask the client to once again use the tiles to spell the thought correctly, so that he is not left with the impression that the thought has to change for something different to happen. Rearranging the letters obviously disrupts the meaning of the original sentence, but this process can also be used to highlight the relatively arbitrary ways our minds produce and arrange thoughts. The here-and-now, physical process of feeling the texture and shape of the tiles and noticing the shapes of each letter can also be emphasized to help counter the more abstract, evaluative, ethereal pull of the thought. And the entire process, as illustrated below, can be used to demonstrate how nonthreatening the letters and words that make up the problematic thought actually are. This dialogue mixes together a variety of defusion techniques, demonstrating how many different tools can be used in concert to help create a context of defusion.

> *Therapist:* "I am a completely screwed-up failure." That's a particularly "heavy" thought. Just watching your face when you said it—it looks like it's a very distressing, very compelling thought for you.

> *Client:* I don't even really see it as a thought. It just feels like that's the way it is.

> *Therapist:* Yeah, the tough ones are like that, aren't they? Well, you know I'm a big fan of looking at thoughts from a different perspective, to see what they're made of. Are you okay with trying another way of doing that with this thought?

> *Client:* I hope it's a good one—it's going to have to be to work here.

> *Therapist:* Okay—we'll see. [*Pours out letter tiles on table.*] We're not going to play Scrabble, but maybe these little guys can help shine a light on that thought. If you're willing, go ahead and spell that thought out with these tiles. Maybe even take your time—notice what each tile feels like when you pick it up. Trace each letter with your finger before you put it in line to help form that sentence.

Client: [*Takes a few minutes assembling the tiles.*] There it is.

Therapist: What was it like slowly picking out those tiles, spelling that sentence?

Client: It was weird. I almost lost focus sometimes on the thought as a whole. And the tiles felt kind of nice, smooth. I noticed a couple of times when I traced a letter that I'd already traced before how weird that letter looked.

Therapist: Interesting. So in the process of producing that thought, you noticed a lot of other things were there, too. Instead of being completely overwhelmed by that thought, you were able to notice other things.

Client: Yeah. The thought's still there, though. It feels a bit different, but it still feels pretty real to me.

Therapist: Okay. Well, let's keep this up for a while, then. I'd like you to rearrange the letters from that sentence. You can change the ordering of the words, form new words with them, or form meaningless strings of letters. I'm going to ask you to do this several times. After you've formed a new "sentence," so to speak, stop and look at it for several moments. And feel free to say how you're feeling, what comes to mind, at any point during that process.

Client: [*Rearranges letters.*]

Therapist: That's an interesting one. A few recognizable words, a bunch of meaningless strings of letters. Go ahead and try to say it out loud, just to see what happens.

[*Client says sentence out loud, stumbling over a few nearly unpronounceable strings of letters. Client and therapist both laugh.*]

Therapist: So I guess we could say that is literally another way of pronouncing, "I am a completely screwed-up failure"— exact same building blocks.

Client: Looks different…sounds different…but yeah, all the same letters are there.

Therapist: And this may sound like a dumb question to ask, but those letters there, those tiles—are they a threat to you? Can they hurt you?

Client: I guess I could choke on them. Choke on my own words—that's poetic. Other than that, I guess they can't.

Therapist: Yeah, and people will joke about eating their words, but it doesn't sound particularly lethal, does it?

Client: No.

Therapist: And that "sentence" written right there with those tiles. Does that define you, define who you are as a person?

Client: [*Chuckles.*] I don't think that sentence defines anything.

Therapist: Right, and let's extend that back to the original sentence. These letters, these squiggles on these unassuming little tiles. Can they really, ultimately, completely define how anyone is as a person?

Client: I mean, as I look at them now, that seems kind of far-fetched.

Therapist: Let's try another one—go ahead and write a new "sentence" with those tiles.

[*Client writes another nonsense sentence, and attempts to pronounce it at the request of the therapist.*]

Therapist: And there's another way of saying it. In fact, if it's okay with you, I'd like to say the original sentence, and you answer back with that one. [*Points at nonsense sentence.*]

[*Both speak their respective sentences.*]

Client: I like the way this one sounds better. [*Points at table.*]

Therapist: Right. And do you see what we're getting at? There's a made-up quality to that sentence on the table. Could there be a bit of a made-up quality to the original version? As in, maybe it's not a simple reflection of reality, but rather it's made up from a variety of experiences, some factual events, some half-truths, some embellishments, and probably quite a few omissions?

Client: I see what you're saying. Maybe it's not such a complete thought, not completely accurate.

Therapist: Good. And there's another thing I'd like you to notice. Those two "nonsense" sentences? Your mind created them. The universe didn't just simply dictate "Thus shall it be," and bam—a sentence that corresponded to absolute truth appeared. Your mind created those muddled-up thoughts, just like it created the first one. We know there was something at least partly arbitrary about how you created the last two. What if there's something at least partly arbitrary about the first one?

Client: It's starting to feel like maybe there is.

Therapist: Good. And one more time, why don't you let your mind reproduce that original thought again. Just go ahead and spell it out again with those tiles. And as you do so, stay present with it—notice the feel of each tile in your hand. Trace each letter. Notice the sounds the tiles make as you string them together.

Contrasting Thoughts with the Present Moment

Our thoughts take us away from the present moment, from the richness and solidity of what we can touch, see, hear, smell, and taste *right now*. Even thoughts that simply describe the physical properties of what you are experiencing at a given moment do not describe what you are experiencing right now. By definition, the words used to describe those physical sensations must come after the sensations.

We spend so much time caught in our heads, carried away by one narrative or another, that we forget how one-dimensional those narratives are when compared to the three-dimensional sights and sounds in the world around us. When you fail to notice the sharp contrast between solid, real, in-the-moment sensory experiences and your vaporous, intangible thoughts, those thoughts seem more real, more accurate than they really are. Explicitly highlighting that contrast can help a client defuse from thoughts, as the following dialogue demonstrates.

Client: And when I think about trying to go out and meet people again, I just can't see it happening. I hardly ever have enough energy. No one will ever want to be around me when I'm this depressed. I don't have any interesting stories, I'm not funny. I'm not good at anything. I remember my dad telling me I'm a loser, and he's right. I am a loser. Anyone who spends time around me will figure that out soon enough.

Therapist: Do thoughts like that come up a lot for you?

Client: Most of the time. I think about it a lot at night, especially, and it just gets more and more depressing. I've even imagined what it would be like to go out and meet people, and it always turns out bad. It makes it even more depressing.

Therapist: So you even run scenarios through your head—your mind imagines going out, and tells you it will go badly. And does it feel pretty real, pretty accurate?

Client: Yes.

Therapist: I can see it on your face now, how heavy, how convincing those thoughts are. I'd like you to try something. As you're sitting there, grab on to the arms of your chair. Notice what it feels like as your hands grab them…the sensations in your forearms as they lay there.…Notice the color of the chair arms. And your mind is going to describe all those things, and that's fine, go ahead and let it do that. And at the same time, don't just focus on the words about what it feels like, focus on the actual moment-to-moment sensations in your hands and forearms, on the actual act of noticing the color and the contours of the chair arms and your hands and arms holding on to them. [*Waits a few seconds.*] This may sound like an odd question, but what's the difference between the sensations in your hands and arms right now, and the words your mind is describing those sensations with?

Client: Well…the words aren't the actual sensations. Is that what you mean?

Therapist: Good thing to notice. I'd like you to focus again, right now, on what your hands feel like as they grab those arms. What they actually feel like, in the moment. Notice those immediate sensations. And then tell me how your mind is describing them.

Client: It feels smooth. I can feel a dull pressure on my palms and fingers. My fingers feel tight.

Therapist: And what feels more "real," more solid, more vibrant—those actual sensations you're feeling right now, or those thoughts that try to describe them?

Client: Well, the sensations. The thoughts are there, but like you said, they're not as vibrant or solid.

Therapist: Yeah. And as you notice those sensations again, as you feel them right now, do those verbal desciptions of these sensations perfectly capture what it feels like to hold on to those arms? Like, exactly?

Client: No. I noticed I even have a hard time finding the right words. It's hard to describe.

Therapist: And notice what our minds do. They offer up verbal descriptions, thoughts, like that, and they pretend like those descriptions are as solid, as vibrant, as real as the actual

in-the-moment sensations. And when you show up to the
moment, to those hands gripping the arms of your chair,
how do those verbal descriptions look?

Client: A bit thin, really. They refer to the feeling, but they're not
fully fleshed out.

Therapist: Good. And I'm going to ask you now if you're willing to
think again about going out and meeting new people. For
several moments, just notice all the thoughts that come up.
[*Waits about twenty seconds.*] And now let your mind do
whatever it wants to, and look around the room. And
notice, moment by moment, what you see…what the air
feels like on your skin…the sounds you are hearing.…Like
before, you'll have thoughts about all those things, and
maybe about meeting new people or being depressed, and
that's fine. And notice, in the moment, those colors, shapes,
objects, and sounds…

Client: It's hard. I get distracted by my thoughts a lot.

Therapist: And that's fine. Your mind is an expert at trying to pull you
out of the moment. Every time you notice it's pulling you
away, look around you. Really look at what you see, feel the
sensations in your body, your breathing.…Climb back out of
your head and into the moment, and experience things first
hand. [*Waits about thirty seconds or more.*] Do you see that
different quality to experiencing things in the moment? Is it
any more vivid or three-dimensional than those times that
your mind pulls your attention completely away?

Client: It is. I just get caught up in my thoughts so often, though.

Therapist: But this is important to notice. Our minds carry us away
like that. They convince us they have it perfectly figured
out, that what they say is exactly what is actually there. And
then we check back in, in the moment, and see a vividness,
feel a solidity. [*Grabs the arms of his chair to emphasize.*]
While your mind has you caught up in there [*points to*

client's head], there's a lot more going on out here. A richness. Your mind is claiming it knows exactly what will happen if you go out to meet new people, claiming to know exactly the kind of person you are. What if that is like your mind's attempt to verbally capture exactly what it feels like to grab the arms of your chair, exactly what it's like to hear and see and feel what is happening moment to moment?

Client: I think I see what you're saying. But I really feel like I'm not good at anything. I do feel like a loser. I've experienced that over and over again.

Therapist: And I know those are very compelling thoughts—I know how hard they grab you. We'll keep looking at them from different angles. For now, as those thoughts show up, come back to the moment again. Notice what your breathing feels like. Notice, in real time, what you see, what you hear…and notice that distinction between the "solidness," the vibrancy of what's happening right here, right now—and those more black-and-white, hard-to-hold-on-to thoughts that keep trying to carry you away.

Conclusion

A variety of different language parameters can be violated to produce defusion. We have discussed quite a few in this chapter, but bear in mind that there is plenty of opportunity for the creation of new defusion techniques within this or any other category.

CHAPTER 8

Getting Distance from Thoughts

As mentioned in chapter 4, the processes of defusion and self-as-context overlap, and techniques that facilitate one process invariably facilitate the other. Adopting a sense of self-as-context, of course, involves noticing the distinction between you and your experiences. While your thoughts, feelings, memories, and so on change from moment to moment, a constant *you* is always there to notice that changing content. This assertion need not have any spiritual or mystical connotation. *You* have always experienced the changing conditions of your life from the same physical perspective. Realizing this experientially can have some distinct advantages. Think of some of the ways you have heard people (perhaps even yourself) judgmentally or pejoratively described: "She is a nervous woman." "He is an angry man." "I am inadequate." "You are a hopeless case." In such cases, emotions, thoughts, or behavioral predispositions serve to define the entire person, and potentially restrict how we view ourselves, our potential, and our next actions. In addition to shaping a more constant perspective of who you are, defining yourself according to the content of your experience can also make your behavior more state-dependent. For example, if you have the transient thought that "*I am* too sad to go out today," you may perceive that thought as a definitive description of who *you* are and what *you* are capable of at that moment, an evaluation that may influence you to act (or not act) accordingly.

Adopting a sense of self-as-context—noticing that thoughts, feelings, and sensations come and go, and that *you* are always there to notice them as changing psychological and physical experiences—can allow you to respond in ways that appear inconsistent with them. When coupled with some sort of behavioral compass, such as ACT's values component, this puts you in a better position to do things that matter to you even when "your heart isn't in it" or your thoughts are not perfectly in alliance. In other words, adopting a sense of self-as-context can give you the flexibility to notice your thoughts simply as *thoughts that you are having*, and then to choose whether or not to act in accordance with them. Taking such a stance essentially results in defusing from those thoughts.

For the purposes of this relatively brief chapter, three techniques traditionally identified as defusion techniques which also have a strong and explicit self-as-context component will be discussed.

Take Your Mind for a Walk

This admittedly odd defusion technique allows you to both notice thoughts as something separate from *you*, and to stay on course toward a valued direction regardless of what your thoughts say about that course. Typically, the exercise takes place in an outdoor setting (or at least out of the therapy office). The client is instructed to engage in whatever activity she would like to engage in—walking in whatever direction she would like, sitting, lying down, and so on. The therapist plays the part of the client's very vocal mind, evaluating or criticizing the client's choices during the exercise, trying to convince her to do something differently, commenting on other aspects of the experience, and so on. The client must listen to what the "mind" says (though she makes the moment-to-moment choices regarding whether to actually do what the mind says) but cannot talk back to the "mind." To make a values component more explicit, the therapist can ask the client to make the walk symbolic—that is, to equate moving in a particular direction or engaging in a particular action with some specific set of actions that matter greatly to her in her own life. For example, a mother who loves her children and values connecting with and being there for them could equate walking to a particular place, or sitting steadfastly regardless of the "mind's" commentary and critiques, with embodying that value. It is suggested that the client's thoughts on such matters be discussed in advance of the exercise so that both therapist and client are clear that there is a genuine value at play, and so that the therapist can include commentary relevant to the value when acting as the client's "mind."

It is important that you get the client's informed permission to engage in this exercise, especially if you plan to use some of the client's more personal information to shape the commentary and critiques you make as her "mind" during its course. The client must be clear that you are not endorsing any of the negatively evaluative thoughts she has about herself, but simply echoing them in order to reduce their power over her. The narrative below provides one example about how such permission could be gained.

Therapist: You remember, we've seen how beneficial it can be to look at your thoughts from a different perspective. And we've done a few exercises in here that helped you get a little less tangled up in your thoughts.

Client: Yes, and they've helped a bit, but it's hard. Things have just been hard at home lately, with my kids, my husband.

Therapist: I know—you mentioned how hard it's been to treat your kids the way you want to. And you've told me the kinds of thoughts and feelings that get in the way. I'd like to try a different exercise, one that can give you some more practice in walking in the direction you want to walk in life, even when your mind, your feelings, seem to demand that you do something else.

Client: Okay—what is it?

Therapist: Well, it's a bit of an odd one, but hear me out. We're going to go outside and take a walk. And I'm going to play the part of your mind. Your job is to walk in whatever direction you want to walk in, regardless of what I say—regardless of what your "mind" says. And I'm going to ask you not to talk at all. I'll be your mind, so I'm the only one that gets to talk. And your job is to hear whatever I say and to walk where *you* want to.

Client: Okay, that is a bit odd. What kinds of things are you going to say?

Therapist: Well, I have a fairly good idea by now of the kinds of things your mind says—the self-criticism, the doubts, the second-guessing—and the exercise works better if things hit closer to home. Would it be okay with you if I said many of the same things that your mind says, with the understanding that I don't believe those things and that I'm saying them just to help you get practice hearing them and doing what *you* want to do, rather than what your mind tells you to do?

Client: Okay, I think I'm seeing the point of this exercise. I think I can do this. But what if other people hear?

Therapist: I'll make sure no one hears any personal information about you. And anything I say if others are within hearing range I'll keep pretty innocuous, so they won't know what we're doing.

Client: All right.

Therapist: One other thing. As you've mentioned, you've been struggling to be the kind of mom you want to be with your kids, to treat them lovingly, supportively, patiently. And I know it matters a lot to you that you do that. So what if we make this exercise symbolic of that? Whatever directions and actions you choose during the exercise, I'd like you to imagine that those actions, those directions, are acts of kindness, lovingness, and patience toward your children. Can you visualize that for a minute? Maybe just close your eyes for a minute, imagine yourself walking outside…notice the kinds of things you see…sort of feel yourself walking…notice the direction *you* choose to take…and imagine that being able to walk in that direction is the same thing as being loving and supportive and patient with Chris and Lisa. And with your permission, I'm going to be your mind and make the kinds of comments your mind might make. Are you okay with this?

Client: Yeah, I think I can do this.

Therapist: All right, let's go. Once we get outside, you pick a direction, and I'll start acting as your mind. And remember—I'm not going to be talking like your therapist, but like *your* mind. I'll criticize, cajole, second-guess, doubt. And *you* call the shots. *You* choose where and how to walk, with your kids in mind, and you go and do what *you* want, no matter what your mind [*points to himself*] says. And remember, this is about walking patiently and lovingly with your children.

[*Both walk outside, client picks direction and pace to walk in, and therapist begins talking as the client's "mind."*]

Therapist: This isn't a good idea. You really shouldn't go this way. You know you can't keep this up anyway....You may be able to do this for a little while, but once your kids start getting irritating, you'll blow it...and after a while, you'll forget how you want to treat them, or second-guess whether it really matters to you. You'll get sidetracked by other things in your life, overwhelmed, and slide back into being inconsistent, impatient with them. In fact, you really should just turn around and head back now. What's the point?...Do you really want to go in this direction, or are you just doing it to impress your therapist? You should just stop and sit down. Seriously....Okay, you've been able to take this direction for a while, but you know you can't keep it up for much longer...

The exercise would continue along these lines for about five minutes before a return to the therapy room to process it. The therapist should ask the client, generally at first, what the exercise was like for her. Then the client can be asked questions such as: Were you able to maintain your direction the whole time? If not, do you remember why you changed direction? Were there any things that I said that were particularly compelling, that hooked you? Did you connect with your value of (being loving, supportive, and patient with your children) during the exercise? What was that like? How do those thoughts that your mind tries to push you around with look now? Did any distressing feelings show up during the exercise? If so, were there times you were able to carry them with you and still move forward?

As you can see from the therapist's comments as the client's mind, you should have a good rapport with the client and have her permission to echo her negatively self-evaluative thoughts. If the client is not willing for such thoughts to be used during the exercise, less personalized thoughts that simply attempt to get the client to change direction or critique her choice of actions can be used. And as mentioned before, adding a values component is optional. However, voicing more personalized thoughts and linking the exercise to meaningful and vital actions in the client's life make its effects more potent.

Thoughts on Cards

When you are tapped into your "inner dialogue," thoughts move so quickly and so smoothly that they are typically viewed simply as reflections of reality. The "Thoughts on Cards" exercise both slows down the process of thinking and turns apparently self-defining, distressing thoughts into a tangible product that can be viewed "out there" rather than being immediately believed "in here." This simple exercise requires a stack of 4 by 5 inch index cards (though scraps of paper will suffice), and can be introduced as a way of slowing things down and (you guessed it) looking at thoughts from a different perspective. The client is asked to write down each thought and emotion, as it comes, on a separate index card, and to lay it on the table in front of him alongside the other thoughts and emotions. Even thoughts that comment on the process (for example, "I don't see how this will help") should be written down on cards. The exercise can continue for as briefly as a few minutes, or for much longer if needed. As a rule of thumb, you should let the client's verbal and nonverbal cues determine how long you continue. If the affect attached to the client's narrative becomes less "heavy"; if the client starts to make spontaneous comments that mirror defusion-related words, phrases, or metaphors you have used in past sessions; or if he gives other signs that he is holding his narrative more "lightly" (for example, he laughs or voices skepticism about the content of his thoughts), these are signs that the exercise has probably served its purpose.

If the client gives such indications that he is defusing from his thoughts, there may be little need to process the exercise beyond simply reinforcing the skeptical observations he himself is making about aspects of his narrative. If desired, though, an acceptance component can be built into an added phase of the exercise. Stack up the used index cards and ask the client to sit in a chair in front of you. State that you will be "flinging" each card, one at a time, toward the client's lap, and that his job is to try to keep the cards (and the thoughts and feelings written on them) from touching him. Prior to flinging each card, orient the client toward what is written on it. The client will likely contort himself in a variety of ways, but some cards will invariably touch him—and all the cards, with the thoughts and feelings they contain, will still be there at the end of the exercise. This can be likened to the client's experience of expending so much effort to try to keep his distressing thoughts and feelings at bay, only to find that they still remain.

Next, inform the client that you will once again fling the cards at him one by one, but that he is to simply let them fall where they will, without fighting to avoid them. As before, he should be told the content of each card before it is thrown. The client can then be asked if he noticed any differences between the two phases. Many different features of the experience can be pointed out by the client or, if necessary, by the therapist. The second phase is easier, since the client does not have to make any effort to evade the cards. The thoughts and feelings are still there and potentially in view, but did they really need to be (unsuccessfully) fought off in the first place? If the client mentions that he still struggles with one or more of the thoughts or feelings, you can pick that card up, hold it at a distance from him, and use a number of defusive language conventions (for instance, "And this thought… can you let these words, these letters, just be there, on their own terms?") discussed in chapter 6 to facilitate more defusion.

Leaves on a Stream

This visualization exercise gives the client practice noticing thoughts as thoughts, and is typically used relatively early in treatment to begin shaping awareness of thinking. It is best for the client to close his eyes during the exercise to help prevent distraction. This need not, however, preclude some conversation between therapist and client at key points, as illustrated below.

Therapist: Okay, so we've talked about how automatic our thoughts can be, about how we typically don't even notice we're thinking. We just assume we're noticing and describing the way things really are. It's easy for our mind to take us for a ride when we do this—to convince us that everything it says is true. So I'd like to do an exercise that will let you practice catching your thoughts and noticing how sticky they can be, how easy it is to get lost in a train of thought. Are you game?

Client: Yes, okay.

Therapist: All right. Go ahead and get comfortable. Close your eyes. And imagine that you're sitting in the forest, on a nice grassy bank, right by a stream. Just let yourself notice as many details about that setting as you can…the sound of the water, what it feels like sitting on the grass, the slight breeze in the air, the trees towering above you. And I'd like you to imagine leaves floating down the stream, one by one. As you sit there watching those leaves float by, notice what you're thinking. And each thought that you have, imagine placing it on one of those leaves and letting it float by. Then try to do that with the next thought, and the next, no matter what the thought is about. Are you there?

Client: Yes.

Therapist: Good. Sooner or later, you're going to get stuck. You'll stop placing thoughts on leaves, and get carried away by a train of thought. When you notice that happening, just tell me something like, "It happened."

Client: Okay… [*After a minute or two.*] It happened.

Therapist: Okay. Can you trace back to the thought that derailed you, and let me know what it was?

Client: I started thinking about picking my kids up at school, and then everything I have to do after that, and how busy I always am at night, and how it's always the same thing, night after night.

Therapist: Okay. "It's always the same thing, night after night." Go back to that stream, and place that thought on the next leaf. And the next thought on the next leaf. And so on.

Client: This is hard—I keep messing up and getting carried away.

Therapist: And that thought—"I keep messing up"—put that on the next leaf. [*Fifteen or twenty seconds pass.*] You might notice that some of the same thoughts keep showing up, or that a leaf comes circling back, or gets stuck. And the thought you have at that point, just put it on a leaf again—let it do what it wants—and then the next thought, put it on the next leaf.

Client: It happened.

Therapist: All right. And the thought you're having right now—place that on a leaf, and the next.

Client: [*About thirty seconds pass.*] I keep thinking about how hard this is. I keep going off on a stream of thoughts. I can't do this very well.

Therapist: And that thought, "I can't do this very well"—put that one on a leaf, and then the next thought…

Once the exercise is over, the client should be asked to describe what the experience was like (a rule of thumb for most ACT exercises—allow the client to share her direct experience before it is molded or reframed by the therapist). Many different aspects of the experience might be brought up by the client or therapist: how quickly and automatically thoughts come, and how they lead to related or sometimes even random thoughts; how easy it is to forget that one is thinking and simply be held hostage to the narrative that unfolds; how you always have the option to notice your next thought as a thought once you've realized you've been carried away. Additionally, the client can be asked if she experienced her thoughts any differently when she was noticing them and placing them on leaves—versus when she was carried away by a stream of thoughts. In the case of the client depicted above, her tendency to criticize her ability to "successfully" engage in the exercise might even be discussed. Virtually no one can "succeed" at this exercise (that is, put every single thought on a leaf and never get distracted from the process). She did no worse or better than anyone else does. Yet our minds are capable of arbitrarily criticizing us, even absent conclusive data that our performance is inadequate. How many other fishy, arbitrary thoughts does her mind produce? Could it be that at least some of the thoughts she takes at face value aren't what they claim to be?

Conclusion

Getting distance from our thoughts can help disarm them, help us start to see that maybe they are simply words our minds create rather than mirror images of reality. We have discussed three common ways of providing this experience for clients in this chapter.

CHAPTER 9

Undermining Verbal Rules and Narratives

The previous chapters in this book have primarily focused on the use of defusion techniques with negative evaluations, particularly negative self-evaluations. In fact, fusion with a variety of different types of thoughts can cause problems for us. It has already been pointed out that defusion can be useful in disrupting harmful narratives we construct about our current experiences, or our lives in general. Though they may carry a good deal of descriptive fact, narratives about who you are and what caused you to be in the circumstances you are in can be dangerous for many different reasons. If your life circumstances are unfortunate, your narrative may frame you as a victim or as unable to respond effectively to life's challenges. A person in dire straits would be well within his rights to view himself as a victim or as ineffective, but such narratives often carry unnecessary limitations and prescribed roles. A victim can view himself as fundamentally harmed, psychologically damaged, even broken. The verbal implications of such thinking cascade out broadly. Imagine a woman who very much values intimate relationships, but who suffered a sexual assault and subsequently experiences intense anxiety, fear, and discomfort in intimate situations with men. It would be easy in this situation for her to think things like, "I can't ever be close to someone again," or "My life is ruined"—and live her life in accordance with these thoughts. Similarly, a man who has underperformed numerous times and faced harsh criticism for it could come to think of himself as a "failure" and end up opting out of meaningful challenges because he "knows" he's not up to them. Buying into entrenched narratives about your life's experiences and their seemingly immutable verbal implications can lead to behavior that is counterproductive, inflexible, and harmful. Defusion strategies can be helpful in loosening the grip of such narratives. An exercise designed explicitly for this purpose will be discussed below.

Verbal rules that either prescribe or proscribe specific behaviors can also cause great difficulty. Such rules are often of great benefit, of course. The ability to do something effective simply because you are told how to do it—perhaps without ever having encountered that situation before—is so valuable that we come to rely heavily on rule following. In fact, your history of reinforcement for following rules is likely so robust that you continue to follow some (or many) rules even when they are not effective. A series of experiments conducted in the 1970s and 1980s (for example, Matthews, Shimoff, Catania, & Savgolden, 1977; Shimoff, Catania, & Matthews, 1981; Hayes, Brownstein, Haas, & Greenway, 1986) demonstrated how reliance on verbal rules regarding how to maximize performance often results in relative insensitivity to real-world contingencies. In other words, the more we rely on rules about how to do things, the less attention we may pay to how well those rules are actually working. Rules are often so helpful that we begin to use them as substitutes for direct experience, attending more to what we are "supposed to" be doing than to the effects of our actions. And many of these rules may be relatively implicit—distillations of what we have been told to do under particular circumstances or verbal echoes of what worked in the past that guide our behavior even when we are not fully aware of what they are. After describing the "Create a New Story" technique that targets problematic life narratives, we will discuss several other defusion techniques that attempt to disrupt problematic rules.

Undermining Verbal Narratives

Create a New Story

This exercise typically takes place over the course of several therapy sessions. The client is asked to write (between sessions) his life's story, complete with relevant facts about what has happened to him throughout his life and how those events led him to the psychological state he is in now. Strosahl and Robinson (2008) offer an alternative, more systematic version of this exercise, in which the client is first asked to write down brief descriptions of bad things he experienced that had a formative impact on his life in one column of a two-column chart. In a second column, labeled "Effects," he is asked to write down the effects each event had on him or his life. These effects could include how he thinks about himself, how he thinks about his life or others, how he feels, how he acts, and how he lives. For example, a male client might provide a description like, "My dad physically abused me a lot when I was a kid." In the "Effects" column, he might write, "I'm angry." "I have a hard time trusting others." "I feel worthless." "I feel like hitting my own kids sometimes." "I work a dead-end job because I'm too much of a wreck to do anything else."

After filling out the chart or presenting the story at the next session (note that this can often serve as helpful assessment information as well), the client is asked to retain all the factual events in the story (that is, descriptions of actual events that led to the listed psychological and lifestyle effects). He is then asked to imagine and rewrite the effects of those events however he wishes. For example, across from the description "My dad physically abused me," he could write in the "Effects" column: "Became more loving toward my own son." "Was able to trust some people." "Found a more acceptable job." The altered outcomes need not be more positive or more negative than the current apparent outcomes, simply different. This can be repeated one or two more times. The process can serve to highlight the semi-arbitrary link between cause and psychological effect, to get the client to consider possibilities not considered before, and to potentially loosen the hold the client's narrative has on his behavior. Sometimes, however, the therapist has to work to realize these gains.

Client: But the first story is true. I can see how the others might have been possible, but that's not how it happened.

Therapist: Yeah, I know. It's hard to imagine a lot of these things not turning out the way they did in your first story. It would be pretty hard not to be angry after getting beaten by your dad.

Client:　Exactly.

Therapist:　And my guess is, these thoughts and these feelings that you have now, that are linked to your dad, are going to be there when they want to. Is that how it's worked so far?

Client:　Pretty much.

Therapist:　And some of these others, like "Feeling worthless"…I notice that didn't show up in the other versions of the story. Could you imagine someone going through that experience and not being worthless?

Client:　Well, yes. That's not how it is for me, though.

Therapist:　And notice there's a distinction between *feeling* worthless and *being* worthless. I imagine that when you feel worthless, you think you *are* worthless. Is that right?

Client:　Yes, well, it's pretty hard to avoid that.

Therapist:　And what if it is just a feeling? I mean, is there an ironclad causal relationship between being abused and being worthless…or are some of the other, alternative outcomes you wrote about here possible as well?

Client:　I *guess* they're not the same.…I think someone could feel worthless and not be worthless.

Therapist:　Even this one: "I work a dead-end job because I'm too much of a wreck to do anything else." I hear you—I can imagine how huge of an impact being beaten by your dad would have on your life.

Client:　It's devastating. I mean, they're supposed to help you, to take care of you.

Therapist:　Yeah. And he did exactly the opposite. And "I work a dead-end job because I'm too much of a wreck to do anything else"—there's a sense of finality there, like that's all you'll ever be able to do. Is there a chance you might be able to do something else?

Client: I guess…I haven't been able to do it yet.

Therapist: Okay. But do you see what I'm getting at, with these questions, with all these different versions of your life story? Our minds are pretty good at definitively telling us what kind of people we are, what we have to do, what we can't do, what the world is like. Pretty good at telling us that because "X" happened, "Y" has to be the result. And some of these things you wrote—feeling angry, betrayed, down on yourself—you know those are there, at least *when* they're there. But some of the others.…What if the whole story isn't airtight? I mean, your mind was able to make up alternative outcomes in the other versions you wrote. Who's to say that it didn't do some of the same with the original story?

Client: [*Long pause.*] I see what you mean. I mean, you're right that just because someone feels worthless doesn't mean he is worthless. And I guess I don't really know if I could hold a better job, at this point.

Therapist: Good. That's all I was getting at. What if minds act like the ultimate authority, but get things wrong?

I Am

The "I Am" exercise can also cut through global verbal narratives, in this case regarding the client's sense of self-identity. (Like the techniques in chapter 8, this one also has a heavy self-as-context component.) The client is asked to write the words "I Am" on the top of a piece of paper, and then list all the different roles and characteristics that define him. Encourage the client to include a brief evaluation of how well he performs a given role. For example, he might write, "a good father, a distant son, a supportive husband, a marginal accountant, fat, not good enough, smart, a fraud, lazy," and so on.

After he has finished writing a relatively exhaustive list, point out entries that are incompatible or inconsistent with each other, as a way of illustrating how minds tend to contradict themselves. Then, ask the client to read each entry to you, one by one (for example, "I am a good father"…"I am a distant son"…), crossing off each entry after he reads it. To maintain more of a human connection, and to help the client connect with all the various evaluations he is reading, have him read them *to* you, rather than simply looking down and robotically reading them from the paper. When the last item is crossed off, ask the client to read what remains—"I Am"—and process the client's reactions. The aim of the exercise is to provide an experiential realization that the items, at best, only provide a partial description of who the client is as a person. The contradictions and partial truths contained on the sheet suggest that his mind is not accurately capturing his identity. In short, he realizes "I am" something beyond what words can capture.

Undermining Verbal Rules

Thoughts and Feelings Aren't Causes

Compelling thoughts and intense feelings are often viewed as causes of the behavior that follows. In this case, two verbal rules (or more) are typically being followed. The first is a generalized rule that thoughts and feelings cause behavior. The second rule involves whatever specific variation of this belief the client is currently grappling with (for example, in the dialogue below, the client is fusing heavily with the rule that anger precludes a potentially productive discussion). This exercise is intended to demonstrate, physically and *in vivo*, how thoughts and feelings do not need to dictate or preclude subsequent actions.

> *Client:* But I just can't get myself to talk to my girlfriend. I get so angry—there's just no way I could go over there and talk it out.
>
> *Therapist:* Yeah, I know. When a feeling is that intense, it feels like it runs the show, calls all the shots. I'd like to try something. I think all of us implicitly assume that our feelings and our

thoughts—particularly when they're strong and compelling—force our hand, make us do what they say. Maybe we could do just a simple exercise to kind of put a foot in that door—to let us take a look and see if maybe it doesn't have to work that way.

Client: Okay.

Therapist: I'd like you to stay seated, and try and convince yourself that you're not going to walk over to that door. A simple action, but see if you can come up with a good argument against walking over there.

Client: Okay, well, I don't really want to walk over there right now.

Therapist: Good. And why not? Tell me all the good reasons you can for not walking over there.

Client: I'm comfortable sitting here. It would seem like a weird thing to do, especially before the session's over. There's really no point to it—I'd just end up walking back to my chair anyway.

Therapist: All good reasons. And let's build on that. You said it would seem like a weird thing to do. Like it would feel weird, kind of anxiety-provoking or silly, to just get up and walk to the door and then back to your chair while your therapist is just sitting there, watching?

Client: Yes, I'd feel kind of "on stage," conspicuous, doing something people wouldn't normally do.

Therapist: So there are those reasons, too—you'd feel…uncomfortable? …anxious?

Client: Kind of anxious….I'd feel "dumb."

Therapist: Okay. Can you focus on that anxiety, that feeling of "dumbness," those other reasons you have for remaining in your chair? Even try to exaggerate them, amplify them, for the next few moments.

127

Client: You're going to tell me to walk to the door, aren't you?

Therapist: [*Laughs.*] In a minute, yes. For now, just focus on those reasons, that discomfort, and see if you can convince yourself that you're not going to—even that you can't—walk to that door.

Client: All right. [*About twenty seconds pass.*]

Therapist: Do you have a pretty compelling case? [*Client nods.*] Good. Now, holding those reasons in mind, and focusing on that anxiety, that sense of "dumbness," get up and walk to the door.

Client: [*Pauses for a few moments, then walks to the door.*]

Therapist: Good. You can come back and sit down now if you want. [*Waits.*] What's showing up for you now?

Client: Well, it was actually a bit harder to do than I initially thought it was. I mean, it's an easy thing to do, but when you trump it up, it's not quite as easy.

Therapist: Yeah, you can even start doubting whether you can do something simple when your mind, your feelings, get involved.

Client: Yes, that was exactly what it was like. And I see where you're going with this, but that anger about my girlfriend is a lot more intense than what I was feeling when I walked to the door.

Therapist: My guess is there are some pretty compelling thoughts there as well. What are some of them?

Client: How could she do this to me? Nothing can excuse what she did. I imagine confronting her, and I think, I'll just fly off the handle. Nothing good can come of it.

Therapist: Yeah. Hard thoughts to carry. And I'm with you—walking to the door under relatively low-pressure conditions is a different thing than trying to reach some kind of a resolution with your girlfriend under those other conditions. And…look what happened in here a couple of minutes ago. Your mind, and some relatively mild feelings, gained a foothold with you. They started to describe—in advance, mind you—exactly what the experience would be like, and started to make you doubt that you could do it. Was the experience exactly like you expected it to be?

Client: It was similar…but no, not exactly.

Therapist: So I wonder, there are higher stakes with your girlfriend, and your mind—and your feelings—are screaming louder at you this time. But what if something similar is at play there as well? What if your mind is trying to convince you that it knows *exactly* what's going to happen, that it *knows* your anger can actually get up and physically prevent you from talking to her in some kind of way that might actually produce some results? What if something similar to what happened here could happen there?

Client: I see what you're saying. I don't know. I'm pretty angry about this.

Therapist: And that anger is making a lot of promises about what you can and can't do, about *exactly* what the process of talking to her will be like. Does it really know all that?

Client: [*Long pause.*] Maybe not.

Therapist: Then maybe we've got an opening here we can work with.

As demonstrated in this dialogue, it is a stretch to compare an act as simple as walking to the door with acting in the face of a highly distressing situation. For this exercise to be effective, you may need to make efforts to amplify the relatively minor doubts and discomfort the client experiences, and honor the differences in intensity between the experiences being compared. The primary goal is to build doubt that the client's mind is accurately forecasting an outcome, and to help him experientially understand that he can act in opposition to his thoughts and feelings.

Reasons Are Not Causes

Repeatedly, throughout our lives, we are asked to give reasons for why we have acted as we have. If acceptable reasons are given, our behavior is often excused, or simply viewed as a logical outcome. Over time, the primacy of reasons becomes internalized. We come to believe that if we have compelling reasons to do something, we are bound to do it, and that, conversely, compelling reasons against an action prohibit it. In fact, while we typically do have one or more reasons for acting the way we do, those reasons do not need to serve in cause-and-effect relationships with what we do next, as the dialogue below illustrates.

> *Therapist:* You mentioned that you got in a huge argument with your girlfriend, and you said several things that were intentionally hurtful. I wanted to focus on this because you said that this relationship really matters to you, and you've noticed a pattern where you get in fights and say things that you regret.
>
> *Client:* I just fly off the handle. It's like the anger takes over and I just attack.
>
> *Therapist:* All right, so it sounds like your mind is saying that your anger is one reason why you said those things to her. What other reasons are there?
>
> *Client:* Well, she said some pretty insulting things to me.
>
> *Therapist:* Okay—what else?
>
> *Client:* I didn't realize this until my last therapist pointed it out, but I think one reason I say things like that is because I feel vulnerable, and by pushing someone close to me away by insulting them, I protect myself from really getting hurt.
>
> *Therapist:* Okay, so your mind is saying anger, her insults, and protecting yourself from getting hurt are three reasons that made you say those insulting things. Any other reasons?
>
> *Client:* Well, my parents were like that when they fought, so that's the way I learned to do it.

Therapist: Any other reasons?

Client: [*Pauses.*] None that I can think of.

Therapist: Well, just so we can let our minds be creative, let's see if we can come up with other reasons why someone might have insulted his girlfriend. Not necessarily reasons why *you* did this past week, but logical reasons that someone could have.

Client: She could have deserved them. She really doesn't, but she could have.

Therapist: Good, keep going. Everything you can think of.

Client: I could have some kind of explosive anger disorder. I could have brain damage, or have been on drugs.

Therapist: Good. And let's try for some off-the-wall reasons—really unlikely ones.

Client: Uh, too much violent TV...sugar withdrawal...posthypnotic suggestion.

Therapist: All right, good. A bunch of potential reasons for insulting her. Some reasons were present, some weren't. Some were far-fetched. What about reasons for *not* insulting her—were there any reasons for that?

Client: [*Pauses.*] I love her. I've regretted insulting her in the past, felt bad about it, and said I wouldn't do it again.

Therapist: And it's hurting the relationship, right—a relationship you really want to stay in? Was that reason present?

Client: Yes—it really is hurting it.

Therapist: Any other reasons?

Client: It's just not nice. I shouldn't do it.

Therapist: Good. And can you come up with some really outlandish reasons for not insulting her?

Client:　Okay. Space aliens are watching us for signs of anger, and will attack if they see them. My mom might show up when I'm yelling at her and give me a spanking. Stuff like that?

Therapist:　Exactly. I want to point out a couple of things here. Minds are very good at making up reasons for why we do things and why we don't do things. They can even make up seemingly outlandish reasons at the drop of a hat. It's like when we talked about how random thoughts can just come up automatically, and we can believe them simply because they are there and because we trust our minds too much. Some of these reasons seem more logically linked to what we do next—like those reasons *caused* us to do what we did. And still, they are just thoughts, right?

Client:　Yeah. But it makes sense that I yelled at her for the reasons I said I did. Not the crazy ones, but the logical ones.

Therapist:　And that's an interesting thought, too—"It makes sense." You also had good reasons *not* to insult her. Am I right?

Client:　Yes, but I don't think as much about them when I'm that angry.

Therapist:　And that's an interesting catch, too. Another reason why— you didn't think so much about those reasons in the moment. And…were they still there?

Client:　Yeah, I guess ultimately they were.

Therapist:　So, correct me if I'm wrong. The reasons were still there, still "in existence," if you will—still *very important* reasons. But they still didn't cause you to *not* insult her. Could it be that reasons, per se, don't *cause* us to do anything, but rather reasons are one way our minds try to convince us that we *have to* act one way or another?

Client:　But those reasons weren't that strong at that moment. I think how strong the reasons are in the heat of the moment matters.

Therapist: Okay, so another reason for insulting her: the reasons for doing it were strong at that moment. And even though the reasons for not insulting her didn't *feel* strong at that moment, are they still good, strong reasons?

Client: Yes.

Therapist: And—take your time, but can you think of a time in your life when you felt strong reasons to do something, but you didn't do it?

Client: Well, sometimes I do that with my girlfriend. I feel a strong urge to yell at her, bring her down. But I don't.

Therapist: Interesting. So you had strong reasons to yell, and you didn't. Those strong reasons didn't compel you to act.

Client: No.

Therapist: And I'm with you—when you feel strong, compelling reasons to do something, it feels like you have to do it. Like you don't have a choice. But look at what we're doing here. Lots of reasons to act one way. Lots of reasons to act another. Your experience of having good, strong reasons to yell at her, yet you didn't. What if reasons are just talk? Sort of logical talk, but not words that *make you obey.* Just ideas, feelings, you have. And the next moment, *you* can make the call as to what you do.

Client: It makes sense, but I get the feeling it'll be hard to act on in the heat of the moment.

Therapist: We'll work on that. But I think the first step is just recognizing that reasons are really just thoughts. We think there's a special status attached to them because it seems logical that *these* thoughts can force us to do things. And if we believe that they can, they play along. But what if *you're* the one who gets to choose what to do, regardless of what reasons your mind is giving you?

Teach Me How to Walk

While it is perhaps a stretch to refer to this as a verbal rule, most of us carry an implicit or sometimes explicit belief that thoughts capture the full breadth and depth of reality, of experience. (If there is an implicit rule at play here, perhaps it is something along the lines of "Words are powerful, so trust them.") This exercise provides an experiential example of how hard it is to capture even the most basic aspects of an experience with words, an example that can be extended to cast a broader doubt on the mind's ability to capture reality. It tends to work best as a precursor to more focused defusion techniques, and a way of introducing the notion that one's mind doesn't have everything figured out.

Therapist: I want to try something. Our minds are pretty good at figuring things out. They've solved a lot of problems for us, gotten us this far in our lives, and because of that, we trust them. We pretty much figure they know what they're talking about, that they understand what's going on, and so we believe them. Does that match your experience—do you tend to believe what your mind says, particularly when you're having compelling thoughts?

Client: I don't believe everything I think, but when I'm having convincing thoughts, yes.

Therapist: And does it feel like, when you've thought about something for a while and kind of reached a resolution on it, that, well, that's how things are?

Client: I guess. If I learn something new later, though, it might change the way I think.

Therapist: Okay. I think that's basically the way most people's minds work. We assume that the things we really "know" [*mimics quotation marks in the air with his fingers*] accurately capture what's really going on. But I'd like to take a closer look at that assumption—to see if our minds know as much as they think they know. Are you willing to give it a shot?

Client: Okay.

Therapist: Good. So we both know how easy it is to walk, right? I mean, for grown-ups like us, with no big physical problems, it's an easy thing to do, right? An easy thing to describe?

Client: Yes—it's pretty much automatic.

Therapist: Right—it looks that way, doesn't it? So let's test this out. I'm going to stand up, and I'd like you to tell me how to walk—to give me instructions for it. [*Stands up.*]

Client: Um…okay. Just walk forward.

Therapist: All right. How do I do that?

Client: Well, move your right foot forward.

Therapist: [*Looks at foot.*] Okay. How do I do that?

Client: Just…pick it up and move it forward.

Therapist: Got it. [*Looks as foot.*] How do I do that?

Client: Use your muscles in your leg.

Therapist: I'm guessing you know what I'm going to say.…How do I do that?

Client: Just concentrate on picking up your right foot and moving it forward with the muscles in your right leg.

Therapist: All right. [*Closes eyes and concentrates.*] It's not working.

Client: I give up—you just do it.

Therapist: Okay. A bit frustrating, I know. But do you see what I'm getting at? Even a simple thing like walking is more complex than it looks. Think about how long it takes a one-year-old to learn how to walk. All the trial and error, learning the hard way again and again how to move one foot forward, shift your weight at exactly the right times, exactly how to place your foot when you put it down, to

135

compensate for uneven surfaces, and all that. A lot of complexity—and yet our minds think it's so simple to capture the intricacies of it. And my mind did the same thing yours did just now the first time someone did this exercise with me.

Client: Okay—good to hear it wasn't just me.

Therapist: And think about that. If our minds can't even accurately describe how to walk, how good do you think they are at capturing the complexity of other things? Like the complexity of your life, of all the things that have happened to you?

Client: Hmm. Not very good, I guess.

Therapist: And to hit even closer to home, since we were talking about how worthless you feel....Considering what happened just now, how good do you think your mind is at accurately measuring your worth as a person? Your worth is quite a bit more complex than walking, right?

Client: Yeah, it is. [*Long pause.*] I guess it can't be very good at it, but I'm struggling to figure out where it's wrong.

Therapist: And I wonder, if I'd asked you to give a written account of how to walk before we tried it, do you think you'd struggle to figure out where *it* was wrong before we did that exercise?

Client: Probably.

Therapist: What's important now is that you're recognizing your mind may not have you completely pegged. It's telling you it knows everything, but that's very fishy.

Conclusion

Verbal rules about how and when to do things, about how and when not to do things, and about how much to trust the "descriptions" our minds give us about our experiences can be very helpful. But when applied too rigidly, with insensitivity to how effectively those rules actually function, they can cause tremendous problems. While several ways of helping clients break the hold of such rules have been discussed in this chapter, many other methods may serve a similar purpose. Something as simple as testing the limits of a "tried and true" rule such as "Always be nice to people" (for example, is this rule prudent and effective under *all* conditions?) might help a client begin questioning the viability of closely held dysfunctional rules. Exploring historical outcomes of the client's following a problematic rule, looking for times when the rule may have led her astray, might prove similarly effective. Put simply, there are no hard-and-fast rules about how to undermine rules.

CHAPTER 10

Assessing Cognitive Defusion and Its Effects

Now that you know how to use a variety of different defusion techniques, you may well be interested in determining how fused or defused your clients are, both moment to moment during a therapy session and over the course of treatment. You may also be interested in seeing what empirical support exists for using defusion toward therapeutic ends. I'll start by discussing signs that imminently signal relative degrees of client fusion and defusion. Then, I'll briefly review two valid and reliable self-report measures that assess changes over time in a client's degree of fusion with his or her thoughts in general. The remainder of the chapter will summarize published empirical evaluations of various defusion techniques.

Signs of Cognitive Fusion and Defusion in Clients

To date, no published empirical studies have focused directly on moment-to-moment cues that indicate a client's relative degree of fusion with or defusion from thoughts in session, forcing us to rely on clinical experience and intuition to determine what these verbal and nonverbal cues are. We can, however, further focus such subjective observations by considering how defusion is conceptualized and letting that conceptualization point to the kinds of verbal and nonverbal client cues that likely signal defusion and fusion.

Signs of Cognitive Fusion

Defusion involves breaking the rules of "language as usual," creating a context where thoughts are spoken and viewed differently, rather than being blindly accepted by the client as simple commentaries on reality. In general, then, a client is relatively fused with his thoughts when he's speaking them "normally," in a manner that would be expected given the content of those thoughts.

More specifically, a client is relatively fused with her problematic thoughts when she is immersed in the content of what she is saying, with no apparent recognition that circumstances could be other than how she is viewing them. In other words, a fully fused client speaks as if what she is saying is simply a perfectly truthful commentary on how things are, without recognizing that she is even having thoughts in the first place. Bear in mind, though, that fusion and defusion occur on a continuum and that lesser degrees of fusion may still require intervention on your part. A client may, at times, identify some of his evaluative or otherwise problematic thoughts as thoughts but get "sucked in" by the content of other thoughts within the same dialogue. In such cases, you may well need to use one of the many defusion techniques discussed earlier in this book. In cases where the client appears to understand the concept of defusion, using simple "mind" and "thought" language (discussed in chapter 5) with the fused thoughts, or referring back to a defusion metaphor or exercise the client resonated with, may be appropriate.

Fusion often coincides with the use of absolute terms such as "have to," "can't," "must," "shouldn't," or other words that prescribe or proscribe particular actions. It also frequently coincides with language that negatively evaluates the client, her situation, people around her, or life or the world in general. However, it is important to remember that the mere presence or absence of particular words or evaluations does not solely indicate how fused the client is. If she shows signs that she recognizes those particular thoughts simply as thoughts (or shows other signs of defusion detailed below), their mere presence would not suggest fusion. For example, a client previously fused with a thought like, "I can't do anything right," might demonstrate a relative lack of fusion if she later stated, "There's that thought again—'I can't do anything right.'"

Conformity with other language parameters discussed in chapter 7 signals fusion as well. A client may be relatively fused, for example, if he speaks about problematic thoughts in a matter-of-fact tone at a normal rate of speech. At other times, the intensity or "being carried away by the story" quality suggested by a somewhat accelerated rate of speech may signal relative degrees of fusion. A tone of voice and nonverbal behaviors that match the affect expected given the content of the narrative similarly suggest fusion. Bear in mind, however, that clients attempting to remain disconnected from their distressing emotions may speak and act in ways discordant with expected emotions and still be fused with associated thoughts.

A final note about addressing fusion with positive evaluative language is in order. This book has explicitly focused on using defusion to undermine the effects of thoughts that are negatively evaluative or otherwise problematic, including those that are unnecessarily prescriptive or proscriptive. Fusion with positively evaluative thoughts can be problematic as well. For example, a client might positively evaluate a current romantic relationship that isn't so rosy after all in a dysfunctional effort to push off of the distress caused by that relationship. A client who positively evaluates himself as a "good dad" might ignore personally meaningful opportunities to act more consistently with his parenting values because he believes he is already doing a "good-enough" job. A client's overly positive views about himself might cause problems in his interpersonal relationships. Or, a client who feels better after doing a defusion exercise might frame that as a "good" thing, indicating that she is still pursuing a primary agenda of "feeling better" as opposed to living in a more values-consistent manner regardless of what feelings are present. You should be alert to potential problems caused by your client "buying into" even positive thoughts. Defusion isn't simply used to "target" individual thoughts that cause problems. It's more broadly used to build a healthy sense of skepticism toward your thoughts so that you can approach them more flexibly and respond more effectively to life's moment-to-moment challenges.

Signs of Cognitive Defusion

Signs that your client is relatively defused from problematic thoughts are, not surprisingly, much the opposite of signs that indicate fusion. A relatively defused client may have a somewhat slowed rate of speech, marked by her use of defusion-related language (for example, "thought" or "mind" language) or metaphors. Displayed affect may not be as intense as when previously discussed in a fused manner, or not as intense as would be expected given the narrative's content. Indeed, the client may discuss her narrative in a "lighter" fashion, as opposed to the "heavy" feel that typically accompanies a discussion of distress. She may even find humor in some of her distressing or otherwise problematic thoughts, or talk about them in an irreverent manner. The client will also show more of an openness to related emotions, since defusion facilitates acceptance. In general, the content of the narrative may look much the same as before; the negatively evaluative and prescriptive or proscriptive language may well remain. But the client will often demonstrate through the use of defusion-related language that he is not taking that content as literally as before. He will also more obviously demonstrate that he is experiencing a sense of self-as-context, putting his thoughts on display as thoughts, and implicitly or explicitly noticing the distinction between himself and his thoughts.

Defusion Self-Report Instruments

Several self-report instruments assessing various aspects of cognitive defusion have been published. Two of these instruments will be briefly described here, and they are included as appendices A and B at the end of this book. The Cognitive Fusion Questionnaire (CFQ; Gillanders et al., 2014) is a seven-item measure appropriate for use with any clients and research subjects. The CFQ correlates well with other existing ACT process measures, indicating good validity, and has good test-retest reliability as well. In a clinical capacity, the measure is perhaps best used to capture changes in degree of defusion occurring across multiple sessions of therapy, as well as to determine baseline levels of defusion in new clients.

The Believability of Anxious Feelings and Thoughts Questionnaire (BAFT; Herzberg et al., 2012), not surprisingly, assesses defusion from anxiety-related thoughts. It also has good reliability and validity, and it can be used clinically in the same manner as the CFQ, albeit only for clients struggling with anxiety.

Empirical Evaluations of Defusion Interventions

The ideal way to measure the real-world effect of a single therapeutic component is to measure it under real-world conditions. This, of course, is the rationale behind using randomized controlled trials to assess the impact of different forms of psychotherapy. To date, no such trials have been conducted using defusion as a stand-alone treatment. Given the description of defusion presented throughout this book, you can probably understand why. While defusion can have some potentially powerful effects, it is likely best used in conjunction with other treatment components, as it is in ACT.

However, defusion's effects have been assessed numerous times in published research, both in the context of broader ACT outcome studies and analogue laboratory experiments. Three of these studies used statistical procedures in an attempt to isolate the impact of defusion during mediational analyses of full-scale ACT outcome studies. The impact of defusion alone has been further investigated in fourteen lab-based analogue component studies, and a meta-analysis has estimated the effects of defusion in numerous analogue component studies where defusion was included as one of several components. These studies, and two correlational studies, will now be summarized and discussed.

Mediational Analyses

Mediational analyses refer to psychotherapy outcome studies where the effects of specific therapeutic processes are isolated using statistical procedures, assessed, and shown to mediate (i.e., to cause) a significant portion of overall therapeutic improvement in subjects. While a considerable amount of mediational evidence exists suggesting that ACT processes as a whole are associated with therapeutic change, it is markedly less common for researchers to assess the mediational effects of a single therapeutic process. Only three outcome studies isolating the effects of defusion have been published.

Hesser, Westin, Hayes, and Andersson (2009) analyzed videotapes of nineteen subjects with tinnitus who received ACT treatment. Trained raters coded thirty-minute excerpts from each client's second, fourth, and sixth sessions for frequency and peak levels of cognitive defusion and acceptance. The frequency with which defusion was used (r = .62) and peak defusion (the highest-rated incident of defusion for each client, rated on a 5-point Likert scale: r = .50) in the second session significantly predicted client outcomes on the Tinnitus Handicap Inventory (which measures tinnitus-related handicap and distress) at a six-month follow-up. Second-session data was reportedly selected because a majority of therapeutic change occurred before the fourth session.

Forman and colleagues (2012) found that changes on a defusion measure mediated a significant amount of improvement in an ACT versus CBT study with 174 mixed anxious and depressed clients, in addition to more generally finding that cognitive and affective change strategies mediated CBT outcomes and that acceptance strategies mediated ACT outcomes. However, the process questionnaire developed for the study does not currently have any published psychometric data, and appears to have assessed defusion with a single question, making it difficult to determine how much of a mediational role defusion may have played.

The most convincing mediational data on defusion to date comes from a multisite mixed anxiety disorders outcome study comparing traditional CBT to ACT. Arch, Wolitzky-Taylor, Eifert, and Craske (2012) administered the Believability of Anxious Feelings and Thoughts scale (BAFT; Herzberg et al., 2012) in each of the study's eleven sessions. They found that changes in cognitive defusion mediated worry reduction, quality of life, overt behavioral avoidance, and depression. Perhaps surprisingly, these significant mediations occurred in both the ACT and CBT conditions, with defusion actually emerging as a stronger predictor of worry reduction in the CBT condition (though ACT produced greater changes on the BAFT scale over the course of the study). This suggests that defusion can be a viable strategy in CBT (and perhaps other treatments), a topic discussed at length in chapter 3. As a possible explanation for why CBT outperformed ACT in worry reduction in the context of this study, it should be noted that within ACT, clients would explicitly be instructed that defusion techniques should not be used in an attempt to reduce the frequency of worrisome thoughts, but rather for the purpose of helping clients to simply recognize such thoughts as thoughts. In contrast, techniques that served a defusive intent in CBT would typically be used with the explicit intent of changing worrisome thoughts. Thus, defusion may have resulted in more worry reduction in the CBT condition because subjects were explicitly using defusion-related techniques for that purpose. (See chapter 3 for a discussion of why defusion could be an active process in CBT.)

Analogue Component Studies

In the context of psychotherapy research, analogue component studies involve the testing of a typically brief implementation of one or a small number of specific therapeutic techniques under scripted and highly controlled conditions. When conducted properly, such studies allow a more precise assessment of what these techniques, and the processes they enact, can accomplish. The downside, of course, is that such high levels of control can result in interventions that are incomplete or artificial when compared to a full course of psychotherapy. The arguable ideal is to conduct both mediational analyses in psychotherapy outcome studies and analogue component studies testing treatment-specific processes, and look for a convergence of evidence.

In the first published cognitive defusion analogue component study, Masuda, Hayes, Sackett, and Twohig (2004) used a word-repetition task to target distress with a total of eight subjects in two successive experiments (four subjects in each experiment) using alternating-treatment single-subject designs (Barlow, Nock, & Hersen, 2008). In an individual meeting with the experimenter, each subject was asked to think of two distressing negative self-evaluations that he or she believed, and then to restate these evaluations using one word each. In preparation for the defusion phase in both experiments, subjects were given a five-minute defusion rationale and then asked to repeat the word "milk" out loud rapidly for thirty seconds to experientially demonstrate the effects of defusion. In the first experiment, subjects in a distraction phase were asked to read an article about Japan for five and a half minutes.

In the second experiment, instructions for a thought-control phase involved a five-minute rationale behind using positive self-talk, positive imagery, and breathing training to change negative thoughts, followed by a thirty-second breathing exercise. Prior to each phase, subjects were then instructed to think about one of their one-word negative self-evaluations and apply any strategy they wanted to try "not to think of the negative thought" (Masuda et al., 2004, p. 480). Subjects were asked several times during each phase how much discomfort or distress they were experiencing on a scale of 0–100, and how believable the evaluation was. Discomfort and believability scores in the defusion phase were consistently lower than in the distraction and thought-control phases. As was previously noted, subjects were allowed to use any strategy they wished during each phase, so it is possible that one or more subjects did not use the strategy they were instructed to use.

In a follow-up study, Masuda and colleagues (2009) conducted another pair of experiments. In the first experiment, sixty-seven subjects were randomly assigned to a five-minute defusion-rationale-only condition (condition 1), a defusion-rationale plus three-second thought-repetition condition (condition 2), or a defusion-rationale plus twenty-second thought-repetition condition (condition 3). The content of the defusion training and other pre-experiment procedures otherwise mirrored the Masuda and colleagues (2004) experiment. On average, subjects in condition 1 reported distress being reduced by 5.1 units on the 100-point scale, subjects in condition 2 by 39.3 units, and subjects in condition 3 by 39.6 units. The believability of the negative self-evaluations was reduced by an average of 4 units in condition 1, 26.3 units in condition 2, and 48.5 units in condition 3. Statistically significant differences in discomfort and believability were detected between condition 1 and condition 2, and between condition 1 and condition 3, but not between conditions 2 and 3. The same significant differences emerged in believability, except that condition 2 produced a significantly less robust reduction in believability than condition 3.

In the second experiment, seventy-seven subjects were randomly assigned to a five-minute defusion-rationale plus one-second thought-repetition condition (condition 1), a defusion-rationale plus ten-second thought-repetition condition (condition 2), or a defusion-rationale plus thirty-second thought-repetition condition (condition 3). All other procedures were identical to the first experiment. On average, subjects in condition 1 reported distress being reduced by about 12 units on the 100-point scale, subjects in condition 2 by about 37 units, and subjects in condition 3 by about 41 units (reductions are displayed only on a bar graph in the article, with no precise numbers provided). The believability of the negative self-evaluations was reduced by an average of 12 units in condition 1, 29 units in condition 2, and 42 units in condition 3. Statistically significant differences in both discomfort and believability were detected uniformly between condition 1 and condition 2, and between condition 1 and condition 3, but not between conditions 2 and 3. As with the Masuda and colleagues (2004) study, a manipulation check was not conducted. Additionally, the three different types of defusion training were not compared to a control condition. However, it is interesting to note that even brief word repetition (ten seconds) combined with didactic training produced significantly better effects, and that the believability of a negative self-evaluation is impacted somewhat differently by defusion than is the discomfort induced by the corresponding thoughts.

As with previous studies, an experiment conducted by Masuda, Feinstein, Wendell, and Sheehan (2010) compared the impact of word repetition and thought distraction on the believability and distress elicited by negative self-referential thoughts. However, to make the results more relevant to a clinical population, only subjects with elevated levels of depression were included. A total of 147 subjects participated in the study, with 71 receiving a score on the Beck Depression Inventory (BDI) in excess of 10, the cutoff score for mild depression. These subjects were randomly assigned to one of five conditions. The partial-defusion condition involved a defusion rationale, a twenty-second word-repetition ("milk") task, and a suggestion that the same task could be helpful in dealing with the one-word negative self-referential thought each subject had generated in a prior portion of the experiment. Subjects in the full-defusion condition received a similar five-minute intervention, but received thirty seconds of practice in repeating one of the negative self-referential words they had generated instead of using the word "milk." The partial-distraction condition involved a thought-distraction rationale. Once a rationale was provided, subjects were asked to say the word "milk" once, then to focus on "all of its perceptual functions" (Masuda et al.,

2010, p. 526), and then to try to distract themselves from thinking about milk by attending to a picture of geometric shapes for twenty seconds. The full-distraction condition was identical except that subjects were asked to focus on the picture of geometric shapes for thirty seconds. Finally, in the distraction-based experimental control condition, subjects were simply asked to read an informational article unrelated to the experiment for five minutes. Only the full-defusion condition produced statistically significant pre- to posttest changes in the believability and distress elicited by each subject's negative self-referential thoughts, reducing them by an average of 37–40 points on a 100-point scale for the entire sample. The full-defusion intervention also significantly reduced believability and distress in the elevated depression subsample, but less robustly, with an average reduction of 26–27 points. Thus, the word-repetition technique seems to be most effective when it is provided with a clear clinical rationale and applied to the actual negative self-referential thoughts that distress participants.

De Young, Lavender, Washington, Looby, and Anderson (2010) compared the effects of the word-repetition technique (WRT) to the Implicit Association Task (IAT) on discomfort and believability associated with potentially distressing words. The IAT involves flashing two words on a computer and instructing each subject to sort each word into one of two categories. Research has indicated that subjects take longer to categorize undesirable or distressing words, so words sorted with longer hesitation are assumed to elicit some degree of distress or distaste. The IAT was chosen as a comparison condition because, in direct contrast to a defusion technique like the WRT, it requires subjects to focus on the literal content of words. Subjects in the IAT condition completed the IAT with four "good" target words, as well as two words they had previously rated as most believable and two words previously rated as most uncomfortable. Subjects in the WRT condition repeated the word "milk" for thirty seconds, then repeated all four "good" target words used in the experiment, as well as two words previously rated as most believable and two words previously rated as most uncomfortable. Two hundred subjects were randomly assigned to five conditions: a control condition, an IAT or WRT condition in which a rationale for the intervention was given, or an IAT or WRT condition in which no rationale was given. When comparing pre- and posttest ratings of the words used in the study, both the IAT and WRT significantly decreased believability and discomfort associated with the words that had been targeted in the respective interventions, with the WRT having a greater effect. Additionally, the WRT significantly decreased the discomfort associated with words not specifically targeted by the respective interventions. There were no differences between the rationale and no-rationale conditions.

In an examination of the word-repetition technique (WRT) with a pseudoclinical sample, Watson, Burley, and Purdon (2010) compared its impact on contamination-related thoughts to a brief imaginal-exposure (IE) and no-intervention control condition (CONT). Ninety-three subjects drawn from a university introductory psychology class who scored at clinical levels on the contamination subscale of the Padua Inventory participated in the study. Each subject was asked to rate a list of nine contamination-related words, then to rank the three most distressing of those words, and then to write a sentence describing a distressful thought they had had involving each of those latter three words. Each subject then made baseline ratings of the believability, meaningfulness, and distressfulness of their words on a 100-point Likert scale. All subjects then completed a combined manual and decision task (CMDT). This particular CMDT presented 116 pairs of either neutral or contamination-related words (tailored to the three words each subject had previously selected and rated) on a computer screen, where one word constituted a category and the second "target" word either fit or did not fit into the category. After presentation of each pair, each subject was prompted to press keys indicating whether or not the target word was a member of the category. Subjects in the WRT condition were instructed to speak each category word one time aloud when it appeared, while IE subjects were told "to imagine a scene involving [each] category word" (Watson et al., 2010, p. 340). The CMDT was included in the experiment to allow an assessment of whether semantic satiation (where words lose meaning after repeated exposure, usually through word repetition) could be produced by the task and whether observed semantic association correlated with changes in later parts of the experiment.

After taking a second set of preintervention ratings on the chosen contamination words, subjects assigned to the WRT condition received a five-minute rationale for the technique, followed by thirty seconds of repeating the word "milk," just as in the Masuda and colleagues (2004) study. These subjects then repeated each of their three selected contamination words for thirty seconds, rating meaningfulness, believability, and distressfulness after each bout of word repetition. In the IE condition, subjects viewed a four-minute, fifteen-second video highlighting the rationale behind exposure and a brief demonstration, and were then asked to imagine a scene involving each contamination word for thirty seconds before rating each word in turn. CONT subjects simply sat quietly for five minutes before making postintervention ratings. Finally, subjects returned a week later to make follow-up ratings of their contamination words. After the three-dimensional ratings made for each contamination word for each subject at each data collection point were averaged to simplify data analysis, significantly higher pre- to postintervention rating changes emerged in the WRT condition, an effect that did not maintain at follow-up. Analysis of data from the CMDT trials indicated that it did not induce semantic satiation.

Part two of the Watson and colleagues (2010) study, which included 134 subjects across the three conditions, largely replicated part one. The only addition involved a request for subjects in the IE and WRT conditions to practice their respective technique for five minutes per day in the week leading to the follow-up assessment, registering online each day after completing this practice. Reductions in ratings for the verbal repetition group were significantly greater than for the CONT and IE groups from pre- to posttest, and from pretest to follow-up. The IE condition did not produce any significant results when compared to the CONT condition. However, ratings in the IE condition improved significantly from baseline to follow-up on the Vigilance and Avoidance Questionnaire, an experimental measure intended to assess awareness of obsessive thoughts and experiential avoidance strategies used with respect to those thoughts. Considering that avoidance was not directly targeted in the WRT condition, and that the notion that one should openly experience contamination thoughts was explicit in the IE condition, the latter finding should perhaps not come as a surprise.

In an extension of the Masuda and colleagues (2004; 2009) studies, Deacon, Fawzy, Lickel, and Wolitzky-Taylor (2011) compared the effects of the word-repetition technique to a brief cognitive restructuring intervention on body image distress to twenty-six female subjects who reported significant eating disorder symptoms. In the defusion condition, participants practiced ACT's word-repetition technique, where they repeated two separate distressing body image–related words for sixty seconds each and observed the loss of word meaning and conviction about the veracity of language that results. Defusion subjects were then asked to use the technique over the course of the next week as body image–related thoughts arose. In the cognitive restructuring condition, subjects were individually led through a thought-record exercise where they identified the negative thought, the situation it occurred in, evidence for and against the thought, and a "balanced conclusion" (p. 223). Additionally, subjects were taught several questions they could ask themselves to help decatastrophize body image thoughts. Subjects in the defusion condition experienced significantly greater reductions in body image concerns, or beliefs about the importance of body image–related thoughts ("fat").

The comparison of brief defusion and restructuring techniques in analogue component studies raises a potential concern. One could argue that the logical and systematic nature of cognitive restructuring requires a more extensive period of time to establish its full effectiveness, and that the brief but potent nature of ACT's word-repetition technique makes it a more ideal candidate for a brief lab-based experiment. Alternately, one could argue that the relatively brief setup that is required to use most defusion techniques could make them more viable treatment strategies. The artificial (though more tightly controlled) nature of analogue component studies suggests that their findings should be taken in context with the results of fully applied psychotherapy outcome studies comparing the effects of ACT and traditional CBT.

Masuda, Twohig, Stormo, Feinstein, Chou, and Wendell (2010) added a control condition to a study that echoed the procedures in the two studies by Masuda and colleagues (2004; 2009). One hundred thirty-two subjects were randomly assigned to a defusion-rationale plus thirty-second word-repetition condition (condition 1), a thought-distraction condition (condition 2), or a distraction-control condition (condition 3). While the procedures in conditions 1 and 3 mirrored those used in Masuda and colleagues (2004), condition 2 involved orienting the subjects to aspects of the cognitive model (thoughts cause emotions and behaviors, negative thoughts cause suffering, and distraction can be used to minimize the negative effects of a thought) and providing them with thirty seconds to practice thinking about other things when the negative self-evaluation was prompted. Results indicated a significant reduction in emotional discomfort between conditions 1 and 3, between conditions 1 and 2, and between conditions 2 and 3. A significant difference in believability was also detected between conditions 1 and 2, and 1 and 3.

In a sample of twenty-two distressed undergraduate students, Hinton and Gaynor (2010) measured the effects of three cognitive defusion sessions relative to a waitlist control. They found large effect sizes in the defusion group in measures of depression (Beck Depression Inventory–II: 1.18), general distress and psychopathology (Brief Symptom Inventory: 1.19), and self-esteem (Rosenberg Self-Esteem Scale: 1.16). As these effect sizes were relative to no treatment, the numbers are perhaps not surprising. However, when benchmarked against group effect sizes for three sessions of supportive therapy (established by Clore & Gaynor, 2010) for depression (approximately .4), general distress and psychopathology (approximately .7), and self-esteem (approximately .8), the defusion intervention compared favorably. These defusion effects, however, dwindled significantly to .41, .41, and .15, respectively, at a one-month follow-up assessment. Such a significant decline could suggest both that three sessions of treatment were insufficient to maintain most positive gains, and that it may be prudent to include defusion as a component of an intervention rather than using it as a stand-alone treatment.

In a nonclinical sample of sixty undergraduates, subjects were randomly assigned to a "prodefusion" group, an "antidefusion" group, or a neutral group (Healy et al., 2008). Before being given a list of ten negative and ten positive self-statements, "prodefusion" subjects were instructed to add the words "I am having the thought that" to the beginning of each statement and told that this would decrease the emotional impact of the statements. The "antidefusion" subjects were told that the same words would increase the impact of the statements, and the neutral subjects were informed that the words would have no effect. All twenty statements were then delivered via computer three times in random fashion, once with the self-statements alone, once with "I am having the thought that" displayed before the self-statements, and once with "I have a wooden chair" displayed before the self-statements. After each self-statement was presented, subjects rated how believable it was, how uncomfortable it made them feel, and how willing they were to read and experience it. For all subjects in the prodefusion group, the defused presentation of the phrases significantly increased subject willingness to read and experience the statements and significantly decreased discomfort. No differences in believability were obtained, perhaps because in each of the defused self-statement presentations subjects were evaluating the believability of the entire statement (for example, "I am having the thought that I am a bad person") as opposed to simply the negative self-statement.

Pilecki and McKay (2012) assessed the differential effects of defusion, thought suppression, and no-intervention on sixty-seven subjects regarding the fear, sadness, and disgust elicited by various film clips. Degrees of these emotions were evaluated using both a 0–100 Likert scale and a standard Stroop task, in which subjects were asked to indicate by pressing computer keyboard keys whether presented color words had been shown in the correct or incorrect order. The Stroop task was included as an indirect measure of distress because prior research has indicated that emotional arousal tends to increase response times. Subjects in the defusion condition (condition 1) received didactic instruction about defusion's rationale and use, while subjects in the thought-suppression condition (condition 2) received didactic instruction on suppression's rationale and use. In the control condition (condition 3), subjects were asked what strategies they use to manage unwanted thoughts, and then given a list of strategies other than defusion or suppression that they could use during the experiment. Subjects in all three conditions were given a practice session in which they had thirty seconds to practice their strategy before being exposed to the emotionally arousing film clips. No significant differences emerged between the three conditions on the Likert rating scale. In the Stroop task, significantly longer response times (suggesting more distress) emerged in condition 3 subjects relative to conditions 1 and 2 after both sad and disgusting video clips were viewed. After the anxiety-provoking video clip was shown, subjects in condition 1 exhibited significantly slower response times when compared to those in conditions 2 and 3. The authors suggested that the film clip chosen to elicit anxiety contained relatively minimal auditory and visual stimulation, which could have made it easier for distraction and similar strategies to effectively function since defusion subjects had been instructed to engage with distressing thoughts when they arose. Regarding the overall lack of significant differences between conditions on the Likert scores and some of the Stroop response times, the authors additionally suggested that defusion is a relatively complex and novel way of dealing with problematic thoughts and that a brief training period is insufficient. The studies by Masuda and colleagues

(Masuda et al., 2004; Masuda et al., 2009; Masuda, Twohig, et al., 2010) would seem to suggest otherwise. It is possible that the word-repetition technique taught in those studies is such a brief and potent defusion technique that it overcomes this tendency, and also possible that other differences in the defusion rationale used between studies could be responsible for the relative lack of effect.

Hooper and McHugh (2013) assessed the effects of a brief defusion intervention in the context of a learned helplessness task. Seventy-four subjects were randomly assigned to a defusion, experiential-avoidance, or control condition, with subjects in the defusion and avoidance conditions given two short paragraphs of instruction to either defuse or engage in distraction and thought replacement (respectively). They were then exposed to a learned helplessness phase where they were asked to choose between two visual stimuli based on criteria set by the experimenter, after being told that the task was relatively easy for most people. All subjects received repeated feedback that they incorrectly responded across all trials. Finally, subjects were asked to complete a maze, using pencil and paper, while being timed. Subjects from the defusion condition completed the maze in an average of 39 seconds, with avoidance subjects taking an average of 52.5 seconds, and control subjects an average of 49.1 seconds. However, since the subjects were not interviewed postexperiment regarding what cognitive strategies they adopted during the maze task, it is not certain what strategies subjects used across the three conditions.

In a very brief clinical intervention that targeted a relatively nonclinical problem, Moffitt, Brinkworth, Noakes, and Mohr (2012) compared the effectiveness of one-hour cognitive defusion (CD) and cognitive restructuring (CR) interventions on chocolate consumption. One hundred ten subjects who reported, on average, craving chocolate at least at a moderate level were randomly assigned to a CD, CR, or waitlist (WL) control group. The CR condition involved a theoretical explanation of restructuring, and instruction and practice on using logical thought disputation strategies commonly used in cognitive therapy (for example, identifying the problematic thought, weighing evidence for and against it, and generating a more accurate thought). The CD condition included a theoretical background for defusion, as well as demonstration and practice of several different defusion techniques, including, for instance, the word-repetition technique and viewing thoughts simply as stories. Subjects were then asked to carry a bag of chocolates for the next seven days and eat them as desired, but to refrain from eating other chocolates. At the end of the week, the subjects returned, had their remaining chocolates counted, and completed a second round of questionnaires measuring chocolate cravings and other relevant processes. Participants in the CD condition were 3.26 times more likely to return with a full bag of chocolates than participants in the CR condition, and 4.61 times more likely to do so than WL participants. No significant differences in consumption were found between CR and WL subjects. Additionally, CD participants reporting high levels of cognitive distress regarding chocolate consumption demonstrated lower levels of consumption when compared to the CR and WL conditions, while no difference between groups existed when low levels of distress were present. Interestingly, this finding appears to be reflective of assumptive differences between defusion and restructuring. Most cognitive models, for example, assume that thoughts and/or emotions must change in order for overt behavior (in this case, chocolate consumption) to change, while the typical assumption behind defusion (as exemplified in ACT) is that overt behavior can change even when thoughts and feelings do not. Thus, for subjects in the CD condition, high levels of distress regarding chocolate consumption served as less of a barrier to behavioral change.

Finally, Luciano and colleagues (2014) tested the effects of a combined acceptance and defusion intervention on avoidance of stimuli that had been previously related with mild electric shock. In phase 1 of the experiment, they used a matching-to-sample procedure to train two six-member equivalence classes using a total of twelve arbitrary symbols and nonsense words (identified to the experimenter as A1-B1-C1-D1-E1-F1 and A2-B2-C2-D2-E2-F2). Next, in phase 2, the A1 and B1 stimuli were repeatedly paired with a mild electric shock (described as "uncomfortable, but not painful"; Luciano et al., p. 97), while the A2 and B2 stimuli were repeatedly paired with points and a display of their current total points. The twenty-three subjects were then informed that, on subsequent trials where they were visually warned of an impending shock, they could press the "Q" key on the computer keyboard (an avoidance response), or the "P" key to earn points and still possibly receive the shock (an approach response). In phase 3, a transfer-of-function test verified that the avoidance function of A1 and B1 and approach functions of A2 and B2 had transferred to the remaining members of each respective equivalence class.

Following the conditioning trials in phases 1 through 3, subjects were randomly assigned to one of three training conditions. Members of the General Motivational Protocol (MOT) condition were told over the course of five minutes that if they did not press the Q (avoidance) key in the next part of the experiment, they would be entered into a drawing to win 5 Euros, a free snack, or other similar small gift. Subjects assigned to the General Motivational Protocol plus Defusion Training (DEF) condition received the same MOT instructions, plus acceptance and defusion training. In a dialogue between experimenter and subject, the impending task was likened to personal situations where each subject was fearful of taking action in meaningful situations, but acted to achieve the meaningful outcome even when at risk of psychological or physical harm. Next, these subjects received a fifteen- to twenty-minute interactive training with the experimenter to "notice and distance from thoughts and feelings as a detached observer" (p. 100). Instructions included defusion prompts to, for example, imagine writing a shock-related thought on a piece of paper, notice the color of the ink, notice whether the words were typed or handwritten, and so on. This acceptance and defusion training continued on to provide several different defusion prompts or techniques, and several opportunities for each subject to practice using them. Due to the ten- or fifteen-minute duration difference between the MOT and DEF conditions, a later condition with new experimental subjects that contained the MOT script plus a ten- or fifteen-minute interactive discussion about issues unrelated to motivation was added. This included subjects first answering several questions about issues in their daily lives, and an eyes-closed exercise where the subjects were asked to imagine doing the things they described during questioning.

In phases 5 and 6, avoidance and approach testing was conducted using both the A1-B1 and A2-B2 stimuli that had previously been paired with shock and points (respectively) and with the remaining C through F stimuli in each of the two equivalence classes. Subjects were again able to avoid shock if they pressed the Q key and to earn points and possibly receive a shock if they pressed the P key. Following completion of the MOT and DEF conditions, twenty subjects participated in a post hoc Control Motivational Protocol (CMOT) condition that replicated the six-phase methodology of the MOT and DEF conditions and used didactic, interactive, and experiential components not related to defusion or acceptance. Further, the CMOT condition matched the length of the DEF condition, effectively making it a more credible control condition. Subsequent data analysis indicated that half of the subjects from the MOT condition engaged in avoidance during both phases, as did about 80% of subjects in the CMOT condition. No subjects in the DEF condition made avoidance responses during either phase, suggesting that the acceptance and defusion training they had received was successful in defusing the avoidance function of the stimuli related to the mildly aversive shock.

Correlational Studies

In a sample of eighty-eight inpatients with diagnosed eating disorders, Butryn and colleagues (2013) found significantly large correlations between scores on the Eating Attitudes Thoughts and Defusion Scale (EATDS) and subscales of the Eating Disorders Inventory (.53 with the drive for thinness subscale; .50 with the body dissatisfaction subscale) and Eating Disorders Examination Questionnaire (.53). It should be stressed that the EATDS currently has no published psychometric properties and that this was a correlational analysis, not a mediational one. However, it would suggest that since cognitive fusion is present to a large degree in eating disordered individuals, interventions that target fusion could help ameliorate correlated symptoms.

McCracken, Gutierrez-Martinez, and Smyth (2013) studied a concept called "decentering" in a sample of 150 chronic pain patients seeking treatment. The authors defined decentering as "the ability to observe one's thoughts and feelings in a detached manner, [as] temporary events in the mind, as neither necessarily true nor reflections of the self" (p. 820); and they characterized it as "consistent with psychological flexibility and cognitive defusion" (p. 820). They found that higher degrees of decentering (as measured by the Experiences Questionnaire; Fresco et al., 2007) correlated positively with acceptance of emotional experiences, values-based action, and daily functioning. Additionally, a regression analysis found that decentering accounted for 8% of variance in psychosocial disability (measured by the Sickness Impact Profile; Bergner & Bobbitt, 1981), suggesting that increased decentering facilitates psychosocial functioning to some degree.

Meta-Analyses

Levin, Hildebrandt, Lillis, and Hayes (2012) conducted a meta-analysis of sixty-six lab-based ACT component studies that included studies measuring the effects of one or more of ACT's six core processes (cognitive defusion, acceptance, contact with the present moment, self-as-context, values, and commitment; see, for example, Hayes, Strosahl, & Wilson, 2011). Six of those studies focused on defusion. Across those six studies (all of which have been discussed earlier in this chapter), a mean effect size of .74 was observed, just short of the commonly accepted large effect size of .8. While that is arguably an impressive effect size, it must be remembered that effect sizes are calculated relative to the other experimental conditions in each study. Some of those six studies included no-intervention control conditions and alternative interventions that may not have had maximally credible components.

Conclusion

While much research on cognitive defusion remains to be done, existing studies appear to indicate that defusion is an active therapeutic process with the potential to produce a variety of desirable effects. Since many of the existing analogue component studies have tested the effects of a single defusion technique (for example, word repetition), future studies should examine other defusion techniques to see if they can achieve similar effects. Additional mediational analyses conducted within psychotherapy outcome studies would be desirable as well. It is especially interesting that the Arch and colleagues (2012) study found defusion to be significantly active in conventional CBT, considering that the intent of conventional CBT is to change thoughts, not to reduce their believability. In other words, it appears that cognitive defusion is relevant and useful not just in ACT and other mindfulness-based therapies, but also in conventional CBT and perhaps beyond.

APPENDIX A

Cognitive Fusion Questionnaire

Below you will find a list of statements. Please rate how true each statement is for you by circling a number next to it. Use the scale below to make your choice.

1 never true

2 very seldom true

3 seldom true

4 sometimes true

5 frequently true

6 almost always true

7 always true

1. My thoughts cause me distress or emotional pain.   1 2 3 4 5 6 7

2. I get so caught up in my thoughts that I am unable to do the things that I most want to do.   1 2 3 4 5 6 7

3. I overanalyze situations to the point where it's unhelpful to me.   1 2 3 4 5 6 7

4. I struggle with my thoughts.   1 2 3 4 5 6 7

5. I get upset with myself for having certain thoughts.   1 2 3 4 5 6 7

6. I tend to get very entangled in my thoughts.   1 2 3 4 5 6 7

7. It's such a struggle to let go of upsetting thoughts even when I know that letting go would be helpful.   1 2 3 4 5 6 7

APPENDIX B

Believability of Anxious Feelings and Thoughts Questionnaire (BAFT)

Imagine the following thoughts occurred to you right now. How valid or believable would each be to you? Please use the following scale. For each thought, please circle a number 1 (not at all believable) through 7 (completely believable) depending on how believable that thought is to you.

1. I need to get a handle on my anxiety and fear for me to have the life I want.   1 2 3 4 5 6 7

2. Appearing nervous is not good and causes me to suffer.   1 2 3 4 5 6 7

3. I can't really do the things that I want to do when I have anxiety and fear.   1 2 3 4 5 6 7

4. I must stay in control of my emotions.   1 2 3 4 5 6 7

5. If I were like other people, I would be able to get a grip on my anxious thoughts and feelings.   1 2 3 4 5 6 7

6. My anxious thoughts and feelings are a problem.   1 2 3 4 5 6 7

7. I am sure to be embarrassed and make a fool of myself when other people notice how nervous and shaky I feel.   1 2 3 4 5 6 7

8. Unusual body sensations are scary and something I need to act on to reduce or get rid of before I can do anything else.   1 2 3 4 5 6 7

9. My anxious thoughts and feelings are not normal.   1 2 3 4 5 6 7

10. Scanning my body for signs and symptoms of anxiety is important to keep me safe.   1 2 3 4 5 6 7

11. When I am very anxious or afraid, there is a good chance that I might be dying.   1 2 3 4 5 6 7

12. I could lose control of myself when I feel anxious or afraid.   1 2 3 4 5 6 7

13. I must do something about my anxiety or fear when it shows up.   1 2 3 4 5 6 7

14. When unpleasant thoughts occur, I must push them out of my mind.   1 2 3 4 5 6 7

15. When I feel bad, I must fight the feeling in order to make it go away.   1 2 3 4 5 6 7

16. My happiness and success depend on how good I feel.   1 2 3 4 5 6 7

References

Arch, J. J., Wolitzky-Taylor, K. B., Eifert, G. H., & Craske, M. G. (2012). Longitudinal treatment mediation of traditional cognitive behavioral therapy and acceptance and commitment therapy for anxiety disorders. *Behaviour Research and Therapy, 50*(7–8), 469–478.

Barlow, D. H., Nock, M. K., & Hersen, M. (2008). *Single case experimental designs: Strategies for studying behavior change* (3rd ed.). Upper Saddle River, NJ: Pearson.

Beck, A. T. (1976). *Cognitive therapy and the emotional disorders.* Oxford: International Universities.

Bergner, M., & Bobbitt, R. A. (1981). The sickness impact profile: Development and final revision of a health status measure. *Medical Care, 19*(8), 787–805.

Bishop, S. R., Lau, M., Shapiro, S., Carlson, L., Anderson, N. D., Carmody, J., et al. (2004). Mindfulness: A proposed operational definition. *Clinical Psychology: Science and Practice, 11*(3), 230–241.

Blackledge, J. T. (2007). Disrupting verbal processes: Cognitive defusion in acceptance and commitment therapy and other mindfulness-based psychotherapies. *The Psychological Record, 57*(4), 555–576.

Bowen, S., Chawla, N. & Marlatt, G. A. (2010). *Mindfulness-based relapse prevention for addictive behaviors: A clinician's guide*. New York: Guilford.

Butryn, M. L., Juarascio, A., Shaw, J. K., Kerrigan, S. G., Clark, V., O'Planick, A., et al. (2013). Mindfulness and its relationship with eating disorders symptomatology in women receiving residential treatment. *Eating Behaviors, 14*(1), 13–16.

Clore, J., & Gaynor, S. T. (2010). Cognitive modification versus therapeutic support for internalizing distress and positive thinking: A randomized technique evaluation trial. *Cognitive Therapy and Research, 36*(1), 58–71.

De Young, K. P., Lavender, J. M., Washington, L. A., Looby, A., & Anderson, D. A. (2010). A controlled comparison of the word repeating technique with a word association task. *Journal of Behavior Therapy and Experimental Psychiatry, 41*(4), 426–432.

Deacon, B. J., Fawzy, T. I., Lickel, J. J., & Wolitzy-Taylor, K. B. (2011). Cognitive defusion versus cognitive restructuring in the treatment of negative self-referential thoughts: An investigation of process and outcome. *Journal of Cognitive Psychotherapy: An International Quarterly, 25*(3), 218–232.

Dimidjian, S. D., & Linehan, M. M. (2003). Mindfulness practice. In W. O'Donohue, J. Fisher, & S. Hayes (Eds.), *Cognitive behavior therapy: Applying empirically supported techniques in your practice* (pp. 229–237). New York: Wiley.

Dobson, K. S. (2013). The science of CBT: Toward a metacognitive model of change? *Behavior Therapy, 44*(2), 224–227.

Dobson, K. S., & Dozois, D. J. A. (2010). Historical and philosophical bases of the cognitive-behavioral therapies. In K. Dobson (Ed.), *Handbook of cognitive-behavioral therapies* (3rd ed., pp. 3–38). New York: Guilford.

Fletcher, L., & Hayes, S. C. (2005). Relational frame theory, acceptance and commitment therapy, and a functional analytic definition of mindfulness. *Journal of Rational-Emotive & Cognitive-Behavior Therapy, 23*(4), 315–336.

Forman, E. M., Chapman, J. E., Herbert, J. D., Goetter, E. M., Yuen, E. K., & Moitra, E. (2012). Using session-by-session measurement to compare mechanisms of action for acceptance and commitment therapy and cognitive therapy. *Behavior Therapy, 43*(2), 341–354.

Fresco, D. M., Moore, M. T., Van Dulmen, M. H. M., Segal, Z. V., Ma, S. H., Teasdale, J. D., et al. (2007). Initial psychometric properties of the Experiences Questionnaire: Validation of a self-report measure of decentering. *Behavior Therapy, 38*(3), 234–246.

Gillanders, D. T., Bolderston, H., Bond, F. W., Dempster, M., Flaxman, P. E., Campbell, L., Kerr, S., Tansey, L., Noel, P., Ferenbach, C., Masley, S., Roach, L., Lloyd, J., May, L., Clarke, S., & Remingont, B. (2014). The development and initial validation of the Cognitive Fusion Questionnaire. *Behavior Therapy, 45*(1), 83–101.

Harris, R. (2009). *ACT made simple: An easy-to-read primer on acceptance and commitment therapy.* Oakland, CA: New Harbinger.

Hayes, S. C. (2002). Buddhism and acceptance and commitment therapy. *Cognitive and Behavioral Practice, 9*(1), 58–66.

Hayes, S. C., Brownstein, A. J., Haas, J. R., & Greenway, D. E. (1986). Instructions, multiple schedules, and extinction: Distinguishing rule-governed behavior from schedule-controlled behavior. *Journal of the Experimental Analysis of Behavior, 46*(2), 137–147.

Hayes, S. C., Pistorello, J., & Levin, M. E. (2012). Acceptance and commitment therapy as a unified model of behavior change. *The Counseling Psychologist, 40*(7), 976–1002.

Hayes, S. C., & Smith, S. (2005). *Get out of your mind and into your life: The new acceptance and commitment therapy.* Oakland, CA: New Harbinger.

Hayes, S. C., & Strosahl, K. (2004). *A practical guide to acceptance and commitment therapy.* New York: Springer.

Hayes, S. C., Strosahl, K., & Wilson, K. G. (2011). *Acceptance and commitment therapy: The process and practice of mindful change* (2nd ed.). New York: Guilford.

Hayes, S. C., Strosahl, K., & Wilson, K. G. (1999). *Acceptance and commitment therapy: An experiential approach to behavior change.* New York: Guilford.

Healy, H., Barnes-Holmes, Y., Barnes-Holms, D., Keogh, C., Luciano, C., & Wilson, K. (2008). An experimental test of a cognitive defusion exercise: Coping with negative and positive self-statements. *The Psychological Record, 58*(4), 623–640.

Herbert, J. D., & Forman, E. M. (2013). Caution: The differences between CT and ACT may be larger (and smaller) than they appear. *Behavior Therapy, 44*(2), 218–223.

Hesser, H., Westin, V., Hayes, S. C., & Andersson, G. (2009). Clients' in-session acceptance and cognitive defusion behaviors in acceptance-based treatment of tinnitus distress. *Behaviour Research and Therapy, 47*(6), 523–528.

Herzberg, K. N., Sheppard, S. C., Forsyth, J. P., Crede, M., Earleywine, M., & Eifert, G. H. (2012). The Believability of Anxious Feelings and Thoughts Questionnaire (BAFT): A psychometric evaluation of cognitive fusion in a nonclinical and highly anxious community sample. *Psychological Assessment, 2*(4), 877–891.

Hinton, M. J., & Gaynor, S. T. (2010). Cognitive defusion for psychological distress, dysphoria, and low self-esteem: A randomized technique evaluation trial of vocalizing strategies. *International Journal of Behavioral Consultation and Therapy, 6*(3), 164–184.

Hofman, S., Asmundson, G. L., & Beck, A. T. (2013). The science of cognitive therapy. *Behavior Therapy, 44*(2), 199–212.

Hooper, N., & McHugh, L. (2013). Cognitive defusion versus thought distraction in the mitigation of learned helplessness. *The Psychological Record, 63*(1), 209–218.

Jakobovits, L. A., & Lambert, W. E. (1961). Semantic satiation among bilinguals. *Journal of Experimental Psychology, 62*(6), 576–582.

Kabat-Zinn, J. (1994). *Wherever you go, there you are: Mindfulness meditation in everyday life*. New York: Hyperion.

Kabat-Zinn, J. (1982.) An out-patient program in behavioral medicine for chronic pain patients based on the practice of mindfulness meditation: Theoretical considerations and preliminary results. *General Hospital Psychiatry*, 4(1), 33–47.

Kabat-Zinn, J., Massion, A. O., Kristeller, J., Peterson, L. G., Fletcher, K., Pbert, L., et al. (1992). Effectiveness of a meditation-based stress reduction program in the treatment of anxiety disorders. *American Journal of Psychiatry*, 149(7), 936–943.

Khoury, B., Lecomte, T., Fortin, G., Masse, M., Therien, P., Bouchard, V., et al. (2013). Mindfulness-based therapy: A comprehensive meta-analysis. *Clinical Psychology Review*, 33(6), 763–771.

Kliem, S., Kröger, C., & Kosfelder, C. (2010). Dialectical behavior therapy for borderline personality disorder: A meta-analysis using mixed-effects modeling. *Journal of Consulting and Clinical Psychology*, 78(6), 936–951.

Koerner, K. (2102.) *Doing dialectical behavior therapy: A practical guide*. New York: Guilford Press.

Kohlenberg, R. J., & Tsai, M. (1991). *Functional analytic psychotherapy: Creating intense and curative therapeutic relationships*. New York: Springer.

Langer, E. J. (2000). Mindful learning. *Current Directions in Psychological Science*, 9(6), 220–223.

Levin, M. E., Hildebrandt, M. J., Lillis, J., & Hayes, S. C. (2012). The impact of treatment components suggested by the psychological flexibility model: A meta-analysis of laboratory-based component studies. *Behavior Therapy*, 43(4), 741–756.

Linehan, M. M. (1993). *Cognitive-behavioral treatment of borderline personality disorder*. New York: Guilford.

Luciano, C., Valdivia-Salas, S., Ruiz, F. J., Rodriguez-Valverde, M., Barnes-Holmes, D., Dougher, M. J., et al. (2014). Effects of an acceptance/

defusion intervention on experimentally induced generalized avoidance: A laboratory demonstration. *Journal of the Experimental Analysis of Behavior, 101*(1), 94–211.

Massion, A. O., Teas, J., Hebert, J. R., Wertheimer, M. D., & Kabat-Zinn, J. (1995). Meditation, melatonin, and breast/prostate cancer: Hypothesis and preliminary data. *Medical Hypotheses, 44*(1), 39–46.

Masuda, A., Feinstein, A. B., Wendell, J. W., & Sheehan, S. T. (2010). Cognitive defusion versus thought distraction: A clinical rationale, training, and experiential exercise in altering psychological impacts of negative self-referential thoughts. *Behavior Modification, 34*(6), 520–538.

Masuda, A., Hayes, S. C., Sackett, C. F., & Twohig, M. P. (2004). Cognitive defusion and self-relevant negative thoughts: Examining the impact of a ninety year old technique. *Behaviour Research and Therapy, 42*(4), 477–485.

Masuda, A., Hayes, S. C., Twohig, M. P., Drossel, C., Lillis, J., & Washio, Y. (2009). A parametric study of cognitive defusion and the believability and discomfort of negative self-relevant thoughts. *Behavior Modification, 33*(2), 250–262.

Masuda, A., Twohig, M. P., Stormo, A. R., Feinstein, A. B., Chou, Y. Y., & Wendell, J. W. (2010). The effects of cognitive defusion and thought distraction on emotional discomfort and believability of negative self-referential thoughts. *Journal of Behavior Therapy and Experimental Psychiatry, 41*(1), 11–17.

Matthews, B. A., Shimoff, E., Catania, A. C., & Savgolden, T. (1977). Uninstructed human responding: Sensitivity to ratio and interval contingencies. *Journal of the Experimental Analysis of Behavior, 27*(3), 453–467.

McCarney, R., Schulz, J., & Grey, A. (2012). Effectiveness of mindfulness-based therapies in reducing symptoms of depression: A meta-analysis. *European Journal of Psychotherapy and Counseling, 14*(3), 279–299.

McCracken, L. M., Gutierrez-Martinez, O., & Smyth, C. (2013). "Decentering" reflects psychological flexibility in people with chronic pain and correlates with their quality of functioning. *Health Psychology, 32*(7), 820–823.

McHugh, L., & Stewart, I. (2012). *The self and perspective taking: Contributions and applications from modern behavioral science.* Oakland, CA: New Harbinger.

Moffitt, R., Brinkworth, G., Noakes, M., & Mohr, P. (2012). A comparison of cognitive restructuring and cognitive defusion as strategies for resisting a craved food. *Psychology and Health, 27*(2), 74–90.

Pilecki, B. C., & McKay, D. (2012). An experimental investigation of cognitive defusion. *The Psychological Record, 62*(2), 19–40.

Segal, Z. V., Williams, J. M. G., & Teasdale, J. D. (2002). *Mindfulness-based cognitive therapy for depression: A new treatment approach to preventing relapse.* New York: Guilford.

Severance, E., & Washburn, M. F. (1907). The loss of associative power in words after long fixation. *American Journal of Psychology, 18*(2), 182–186.

Shimoff, E., Catania, A. C., & Matthews, B. A. (1981). Uninstructed human responding: Sensitivity of low-rate performance to schedule contingencies. *Journal of the Experimental Analysis of Behavior, 36*(2), 207–220.

Spradlin, S. E. (2002). *Don't let your emotions run your life: How dialectical behavior therapy can put you in control.* Oakland, CA: New Harbinger.

Stoddard, J. A., & Afari, N. (2014). *The big book of ACT metaphors.* Oakland, CA: New Harbinger.

Strosahl, K., & Robinson, P. (2008). *The mindfulness and acceptance workbook for depression.* Oakland, CA: New Harbinger.

Watson, C., Burley, M. C., & Purdon, C. (2010). Verbal repetition in the reappraisal of contamination-related thoughts. *Behavioural and Cognitive Psychotherapy, 38*(3), 337–353.

Wells, A. (2008). *Metacognitive therapy for anxiety and depression.* New York: Guilford.

Williams, A., Van Ness, P., Dixon, J., & McCorkle, R. (2012). Barriers to meditation by gender and age among cancer family caregivers. *Nursing Research, 61*(1), 22–27.

Wilson, K. G., & DuFrene, T. (2009). *Mindfulness for two.* Oakland, CA: New Harbinger.

Wilson, K. G., & Murrell, A. (2004). Values work in acceptance and commitment therapy: Setting a course for behavioral treatment. In S. Hayes, V. Follette, & M. Linehan (Eds.), *Mindfulness and acceptance: Expanding the cognitive-behavioral tradition.* New York: Guilford.

John T. Blackledge, PhD, is associate professor in the department of psychology at Morehead State University in Morehead, KY, where he actively researches acceptance and commitment therapy (ACT) with his students. He has authored over two dozen books, and book chapters on ACT and relational frame theory (RFT).

Index

L

M

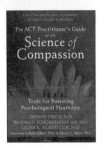
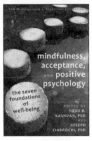
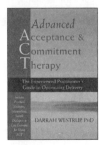
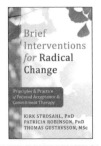
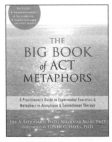
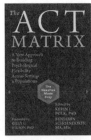